Best wishes
Gerry

SUPER-FIT for BUSINESS

SUPER-FIT for BUSINESS

by
GRAHAM PRICE
and
GERRY RICKARDS

SCOPE BOOKS LIMITED SANDFORD HOUSE
KINGSCLERE NEWBURY BERKSHIRE

First published November 1983

Scope Books Limited
3 Sandford House, Kingsclere,
Newbury, Berkshire RG15 8PA

British Library Cataloguing in Publication Data

Price, Graham
Super-fit for business
1. Physical fitness
I. Title II. Rickards, Gerry
613'.7'1 RA781

ISBN 0 906619 14 9

Jacket design by Janet Lobban
Produced through Print Production Services, Baughurst, Hampshire
Printed and bound in Great Britain by Pitman Press, Bath

ACKNOWLEDGEMENTS

The authors would like to thank the following friends, colleagues and family for their help and forebearance.

David Hughes and Jackie Appleby for being patient and extremely professional models and Patricia Wapples for undertaking the typing. The contribution on orienteering was submitted by Rob Allison, who is a practising expert in that field.

A thank-you to Powersport International and the Medical Centre for their guidance and help.

Finally, to our wives.

Contents

Introduction
Gives a picture of normal executive lifestyle and pinpoints the obvious potential health hazards. Warning signals to watch for.

I **Fitness Problems** 10
A close look at some of the more common symptoms of a business life: stress, over-indulgence, high blood pressure, rapid fatigue and breathlessness, aches and pains, loss of energy and lack of flexibility. Particular exercises to help each problem will be indicated.

II **Fitness Assessment – A Ready Reckoner** 23
A ready reckoner to gauge each person's fitness level in his/her age group.

III **How to Proceed** 32
Some dos and don'ts to observe if you decide to embark on the programme. Some ways to keep up enthusiasm and where to proceed with caution.

IV **Fitness Programme** 41

- ☆ Explains the different body types and how they affect performance.
- ☆ A general fitness programme which includes — pre-stretch, flexibility, aerobics, power and post-stretch. Also including the preparatory warm-up and a series of exercises for the problems identified in earlier chapters.
- ☆ Explanation of how you can carry on the programme at home, in the office and in the hotel. Also some helpful comments on executive travel.
- ☆ An analysis of the exercises for back and posture troubles and problems arising from stress.

V **Par for the Course — How Do You Rate?** 120

A method of comparing your progress with other colleagues in the same age group with a series of balanced exercises.

VI **Case Studies** 121

An examination of the effect of the fitness programme on two selected executives — a thirty-eight year old man and a forty-one year old woman.

VII **How Can the Company Help?** 132

Describes the equipment and space required for a company gymnasium and shows some of the ways a company can encourage participation in a fitness programme.

VIII **The Crossroads** 136
Now you are fit — do you stop or go on? A brief look at an extended programme, specialist activities, recreational pursuits and the martial arts.

IX **Relief of Boredom** 173
A few hints on how to relieve boredom in the day-to-day fitness programme.

X **Microcomputers** 177
How to design a computer application for the executive and the professional supervisor in the modern gymnasium.

APPENDICES

1. Fitness Facts and Fallacies
2. Dietary Considerations
3. Equipment Portfolio –
   Personal
   Gymnasia
4. Sports Injuries and Their Treatment
5. Questionnaires
   Fitness
   Training Programme
6. Training Log
7. Preventive Medicine – A Practical Reality

PUBLISHER'S FOREWORD

We, the publishers, are particularly happy to be asked to bring out this book aimed at executive fitness.

We are well aware that a great deal has been written and spoken lately about fitness, exercises, work-outs, aerobics, diet, etc. This book however, is specifically for the business man and business woman who have particular problems with regard to health and fitness built into their life style, which no-one else except another business man can understand. Therefore, if you are such a person, this book, written by a business man together with an executive fitness expert, is ideally designed for you.

The programmes recommended in this book are not just theory, but have been worked out over several years with the executives of a large multi-national organisation and have been proved to be not only beneficial to the individual participants but also to the company as, among other advantages, absenteeism has dropped sharply among those participating.

The authors are convinced that once you have become fit, by following the suggested programme, you will feel so wonderfully well that you will never again allow yourself to slip back into the old ways. Because, when you are fit your mind is more alert, you feel better physically and you can tackle anything which comes your way with more confidence and vigour. A useful spin-off is that you are still fit and well and confident even when you reach retiring age and will be better able to handle this sometimes traumatic situation.

The pace of technological change is such that only the fittest will survive – all the more reason to make sure YOU are the one at the top.

ABOUT THE AUTHORS

Graham Price, Director of Management Services for Rank Xerox, is well-qualified to put the executive's point of view in *Super-fit for Business.* A Welshman, former rugby player and university boxing champion, Graham has travelled in the Americas, the Middle East and Europe. He and his wife Pamela have one son, Lawton, who is 21. They enjoy good food and wine, and entertaining: Graham savours a fine cigar. Weekends are spent on the West Country farm, but Graham's enthusiasm for fishing and rough shooting have met firm opposition from conservationist Pamela. He took an honours degree in Economics at Swansea and studied post-graduate business at the L.S.E. on a Ford (Dagenham) Trust scholarship. Commissioned in the Army during National Service, he then worked in finance for Ford, Philips and Hoover. His fifteen years with Rank Xerox have included four with the parent Xerox Corporation in the United States.

Gerry Rickards saw active service as a Royal Naval physical training instructor in the Atlantic, Mediterranean and the Far East. He taught physical education in public and prep. schools, specialising in the martial arts and swimming. A qualified Remedial Gymnast, with distinctions in Body Mechanics and Exercise Therapy, he has worked at hospitals and rehabilitation units on neurological disability and sports medicine. Gerry and his wife Irene have two daughters and three granddaughters. Graecophile and extrovert, Gerry enjoys 'a drink, a party and the occasional cigar' and confesses to a 'dislike of fitness fanatics'. His old naval hobby of making ships in bottles has been extended to include modelling buildings and even horse-drawn vehicles in bottles. Gerry has travelled widely, and lectures regularly on fitness, Judo and unarmed combat. Since 1974 he has worked for Rank Xerox, setting up and then co-ordinating internationally the type of programme described in *Super-fit for Business.*

Introduction

All work and no play! . . .

The average executive has a different interpretation of play from that of the authors.

Firstly, there are those who believe they do not have time to devote to fitness because of business pressures.

Secondly, recreation for many can range from the occasional game of golf or squash to playing with the kids at the weekend.

Thirdly, the lunchtime chit-chat, the office party, dinner at the club, after-office hours drinks or an evening's television viewing may be considered as relaxation by significant numbers of people.

How does one strike a balance?

Despite the obvious pressures that executives are exposed to, they normally feel comfortable with the familiar environment which by and large ignores potential and significant health hazards. It is quite obvious that well-established practices cannot be changed overnight – nor should they be. But a rigorous appraisal of the priorities in work practices and lifestyle may mean a gradual shift in the inbuilt inertia. The conclusion is that there is no need to 'throw the baby away with the bath water'. The wind of change augurs well for the individual. It is interesting to note that despite the explosive growth in the awareness of individual health and well-being in recent years, not a single executive of the 230 monitored for the programme in this book had previously achieved the 'norm' within their respective age groups.

The authors find this even more surprising because executives have spent many decades attempting to perfect business processes, organisations, communications devices and latterly robotics by studying bodily functions (*Cybernetics*). There is precious little evidence of the application of business performance standards, goals and objectives to pursuing individual executive all round fitness.

Why should this be?

In general the individual and collective approach towards health is defined as corrective rather than preventive action. The corrective attitude is primarily historical and emulates our work ethic and the 'only visit the doctor if you are sick' syndrome. This approach takes no account of one's general state of health and how this can be improved. For those who participate in annual health screening, it may well be an improvement, but the direction is broadly corrective. All too often there is little attention directed towards preventive methods to achieve fitness.

Commercial offerings and the media abound with constructive ways on how individuals can improve their health. There are a plethora of diets to assist slimming; government warnings on the hazards of smoking; sports such as squash, karate, judo, tennis and badminton; health clubs are on the increase and marathon running the vogue. It is exceedingly difficult for an individual, picking carefully through the vast variety of advice, to choose what is exactly right for him (or her).

How does the individual determine how to proceed?

The first aim of this book is to assist individuals to determine their level of fitness as an essential prerequisite to embarking on a tailor-made programme to improve health, well-being and fitness.

A great deal of emphasis will be placed on self-analysis in order to assess how you compare with a predetermined 'norm'. Following on from this will be a programme to demonstrate day-to-day improvements towards an ideal.

What should the approach be?

Once the initial survey has been accomplished with professional supervision it is important that individuals adhere to the programme and the counsel given.

Going it alone could well set up the stresses and strains that the programme has been carefully planned to avoid. The approach of the individual should be cautiously optimistic – with an open mind for participation leading towards a well-balanced lifestyle of his or her personal choice. The programme can be pursued in many ways. At home, either alone or with the family group, perhaps with the assistance of home video or inexpensive equipment that is recommended in the book. At the office, depending on how much the company is prepared to get involved. At the club where the necessary equipment and facilities are provided.

Who is the programme directed towards?

The programme is primarily directed towards the company executive, simply because a great deal of the research has been undertaken with him and her. Naturally, typists, secretaries and terminal operators have been part of the programme and specific aspects of their problems are covered later in the book.

It is well-proven that participation in a balanced programme of exercise, diet and work can certainly enhance productivity. This is shown in reduced days off through fewer health problems, greater effectiveness and increased morale. An extremely important aspect of this book is how the company can support the employees in achieving fitness. It is essential to procure the correct professional advice before embarking on a company programme.

What is the problem?

Most executives will readily admit to long anti-social hours, extended travel schedules, over-long meals at lunch and evening times, spending interminable hours at meetings, lack of time with the family, peer and hierarchical pressures, and periodic 'social' drinking at conferences, mealtimes and at the local. It really does seem astounding that the average executive considers this lifestyle quite normal and does not realise he is manufacturing a 'timebomb' which could blow at any time unless something is done to redress the balance of the day-to-day 'routine'.

The hurly-burly of business life is the main contributory cause of the following problems which plague the company executive:

- Stress
- Worry
- Obesity
- High Blood Pressure
- Rapid fatigue including breathlessness
- Aches and Pains
- Loss of Energy
- Lack of flexibility

All too readily executives identify with the causes but rarely will admit to the results outlined above. Some occasionally admit to the off day, age or a domestic crisis but as to a serious health hazard, never - they just haven't got the time. An observation from a colleague, friend or family member will sometimes make one pause and think carefully about some of the problems. The oversize problem and the inability to keep up with the children at weekends will frequently urge people to consider a fitness programme.

Each of the problems listed will now be analysed.

CHECKLIST

1. Can you devote twenty minutes to exercise daily?
2. Do you want to be fit for work and recreation?
3. Do you allow adequate time for relaxation?
4. Can you identify with the causes?
5. Would you like an individual fitness programme?
6. Have you the right mental attitude to proceed?
7. Do you suffer from any of the problems listed?
   - Stress
   - Obesity
   - High blood pressure
   - Rapid fatigue
   - Aches and pains
   - Loss of energy
   - Lack of flexibility

I

Fitness Problems

Stress

Stress can result from abnormal factors either at work, at home or pursuing extra curricular activities, or a combination of all of these. The manifestation of these abnormal factors can lead to emotional, mental or physical stress.

Normally, stress is at its most manageable level where the situation is fun and is not perceived as routine, drudgery or without any sort of satisfaction. In the initial stages of any pursuit there is the challenge which does not involve commitment or responsibility to deliver – the idyllic honeymoon period. The stark reality of the long haul sets up stresses and concerns.

Stress appears to be caused by abnormal overload at one extreme, and the total absence of work pressure on the other. Naturally, there are gradations between each end of the spectrum.

The examples of abnormal overload on the executive can be associated with the cyclical parts of the business such as product launches, daily, weekly or monthly deadlines, impossible targets, heavy travel schedules, interminable meetings, the annual planning process. Depending which function an executive operates in, the pressures and timeframe vary. Apart from the normal business process there are the demands of one's peers and superiors to cope with. Pressures external to the business also polarise issues and set up stress.

The stress set up by lack of work and lack of direction can sometimes be more stressful than the overload problems. There is a gradual build-up of frustration and resentment at not achieving a level of satisfaction for a job well done, which most executives constantly desire. The routine mundane jobs can also be stress-loaded. There is a 'norm' and a desired balance at home, work or on extra curricular activities that will restrict stress to a minimum. Any departure from this 'norm' will set up stress which will impair productivity and morale, often significantly.

Although the sources of stress are many and varied, the response differs, depending on temperament, personality and certain environmental factors.

Whatever the sources of stress are, a person who is exposed to stress will go through the following stages:

First, the initial alarm or shock stage. This triggers the sympathetic nervous system supported by the hormone adrenalin causing certain physiological changes to take place. These are clearly recognisable as increase in the heart rate, heavy perspiration, a raised blood pressure, dilation of the blood vessels both in the heart and muscles. In addition, there may be dryness of the mouth.

Second, the individual strives, through conscious control, to adjust the alarm reaction.

Finally, the exhaustion stage. During this stage there can be constant raised blood pressure, irritability, frustration, depression, apathy and/or violent mood swings ranging from euphoria to lethargy with an overriding feeling of insecurity.

Long and sustained exposure to the first two stages, without removing or treating the causes can lead into the third stage when individuals could well need assistance to counteract the long term effects of sustained stress. The ability to identify the cause and the symptoms is the key to the solution.

The fitness programme will describe some of the exercises to counteract stress. These include:

- Relaxation techniques
- Hard physical activity

Over-Indulgence

Over-indulgence, which has been used as a catch-all phrase, results in obesity and its related problems.

The executive lifestyle provides all the necessary opportunities for over-indulgence if one so desires. Part of the perks of the job?

It is quite rare for an individual to pause and take stock of his lifestyle, or indeed even question it. Peer pressure, custom and practice often determine the style. Everyone partakes of the traditional lunch, perhaps enhanced when entertaining visitors or when travelling. The 'joiners and leavers' parties, conferences, working parties, with the associated food and drink, all swell the calorie intake. The odd drink at the airport, in-flight meals, business dinners on arrival, a social cocktail on departure. Whichever way one wants to conduct business there are certain conventions that are difficult to avoid and are normally fattening. For the more unfortunate executives some companies insist on a personal drinks cabinet, cigarettes, cigars and the like. It may be difficult to avoid having a meal with family or friends on the odd free nights.

Naturally, recreational activity, week-end gardening or playing with the children at weekends, tend to counterbalance, in part, the excesses that have built up during the week. However, the self-analysis and fitness tests will reveal how far over-indulgence has taken its toll. It is the sedentary occupation plus this lifestyle that is one of the primary causes of common debilitating illnesses.

There is overwhelming evidence that obesity lowers life expectancy, which is reflected in actuarial tables and the premiums charged by insurance companies. In addition, many authorities are convinced that over-indulgence can lead to heart disorders, high blood pressure, arthritic joints, structural foot defects and many other skeletal disorders.

Apart from the executive lifestyle, many people start their obese habits early in life and find great difficulty in controlling excessive eating and drinking habits later on. The balance between an appropriate calorie intake and activity often eludes the individual. Yet, neither exercise nor diet on its own establishes an optimum metabolism.

Dieting alone seldom works, as not only fat is reduced but also muscle tissue. It is also well known that when you eat and take in more calories than are expended over a period of time then the added weight will be almost entirely fat with little or no muscle being reconstituted. It is essential that overweight people establish and determine their correct balance between energy expenditure and calorie intake. Many executives observe that they weigh many kilos more than they did at twenty-one, evidenced by the fact that their collar size has enlarged by 1 to 1½ inches, their belt has gone out a notch or four, their suits are rather more expansive (can't get into the dress uniform any-more?); all this despite the fact that they may eat less. Not only has drink been left out of the equation but, on further probing, it becomes obvious that the walk or run to the bus, enforced sports at school, village soccer, rugger or cricket used to have an effect. The demands of marriage, the job and other activities have upped the drinking and reduced the activity. The truth on eating is probably a little less at any one time, but more often. The message is simple and clear, the more you eat the more physically active you have to be to maintain a balance. A note of caution at this juncture for the 'greyhound' breed, those slim individuals who boast and honestly believe they can eat as much as they like without a great deal of activity. They may be fortunate in possessing a high metabolic rate that burns up calories quickly, but they may still be obese in terms of the lipids that line the heart, kidneys and blood vessels.

The usual executive lifestyle is acceptable in moderation, provided that adequate time is devoted to daily exercise or recreational activity to redress the balance.

High Blood Pressure

High blood pressure is often associated with the executive lifestyle which, if one looks at some of the contributory factors, is not all that surprising.

Prolonged mental stress, obesity, high cholesterol levels, and cigarette smoking, are some of the more obvious. Other causes which must be considered are, a high salt intake and metabolic factors, and perhaps the most important is heredity.

High blood pressure will, if unchecked, ultimately result in reduced efficiency of all bodily systems, and degeneration of tissue. Reduction or slowing of blood flow due to abnormal blood pressure may result in deterioration of both mental and physical efficiency. In addition, temperature control can be impaired causing coldness of the extremities with swelling and discomfort. Because of the slowing down of the healing processes, any trauma affecting the tissues carries more serious implications. The results of oxygen starvation due to impaired circulation are readily observed in symptoms of rapid fatigue inducing sleepiness or even loss of consciousness.

Furthermore, the metabolism becomes sluggish, which may result in the build up of body fat and inefficient bowel movement.

Lack of sufficient exercise, over-indulgence, and stress may give rise to fatty and metabolic calcium deposits with diminished blood vessel elasticity, and this will inevitably cause high blood pressure. There is evidence to suggest that regular exercise will not only help to control blood pressure rises in stressful situations, but will slow down the rises expected with increasing age.

What is blood pressure?

It is the force by which the blood distends the blood vessels during its passage through them. Measurement of the tension imposed upon the blood vessel walls will determine:

- The force of the heart contraction
- Peripheral blood vessel resistance
- Elasticity of arteries
- Blood volume

There are two pressures of major concern.

First, the pressure of high volume when the heart contracts.

Second, the pressure during the resting phase of the heart. This latter pressure is considered the more important because if this is high, even though the volume of blood flow is low, it may indicate a loss of elasticity in the blood vessels, or perhaps partial narrowing.

Age 20 ideal levels 120/80. It should be noted that the 120 equals the heart pumping pressure whereas the 80 is the resting pressure.

Age	1 *Ideal Levels*	2 *Raised*	3 *Seek Advice*	4 *Treatment*
20	120/80	125/85	130/90	135/95
25	122/81	127/86	135/95	140/100
30	123/82	130/90	140/98	145/105
35	124/83	132/93	145/102	150/110
40	126/84	135/95	150/105	155/115
45	128/85	140/98	155/110	158/120
50	130/86	140/98	155/110	158/120
55	132/87	140/98	155/110	158/120
60	135/89	140/98	155/110	158/120
65	140/92	140/98	155/110	158/120

TABLE 1

These levels are only a general guide and should not influence your decision to seek medical advice when in doubt.

On the other hand, athletes often show a high pressure during the pumping phase especially following periods of exercise.

It should be noted that there are many situations which can give rise to an inaccurate blood pressure reading. For example, emotional states such as excitement, fear or anxiety. It is recommended that more than one reading is recorded.

Where does one fit into the 'league table'? If in doubt seek expert advice. The measurements indicated in the previous table are in millimetres of mercury on a scale.

The indications are as Table 1

Low blood pressure is not generally of great significance, unless accompanied by illness. Some people have abnormally low blood pressure, which may be hereditary. Low blood pressure due to shock, trauma, severe burns or impaired heart muscle contraction are beyond the scope of this book.

It is important to realise that the volume of blood circulating around the body is directly connected to the demands. The adequacy of supply to demand depends upon the efficiency of the heart and blood vessels.

The fitness programme, which will be tailor-made for every individual should they decide to participate, will inevitably optimise the supply/demand relationship referred to above.

Rapid Fatigue and Breathlessness

This may have many causes including anaemia, some forms of diabetes, and illnesses affecting the heart, lungs and blood vessels. But in the absence of these more sinister causes it may simply be due to lack of general fitness. Among the more common reasons for rapid fatigue are, breathlessness due to cigarette smoking, obesity, poor musculature and environmental factors such as air pollution.

Executives may, because of their daily routine, experience some, or all of these fundamental factors. For example, daily commuting in heavy traffic, over-indulgence causing obesity, heavy cigarette smoking, and lack of physical activity. To counteract or minimise the 'effect', appropriate exercise of the lungs, heart and muscles is essential.

The limiting factor in physical endurance is the oxygen supply; by improving the heart's output, the lungs' ventilation, the blood vessels' elasticity, and the power and efficiency of the muscles, fatigue levels are delayed. There is a threshold of physical activity below which there is a rapid deterioration of the body's ability to transport oxygen to the working muscles; this results in rapid fatigue.

The message is clear; regular exercise will improve capacity to endure physical work. In summary, fatigue is tiredness, lack of energy or lethargy. These factors are normally associated with:

- A virus infection
- Anxiety
- Depression
- Tension

Apart from a virus infection which will need expert attention, the executive experiencing anxiety, depression or tension will benefit substantially from the fitness programme.

In the early stages of the programme it is important to get adequate rest and relaxation to avoid fatigue. Pushing up the activity rate too quickly and going it alone can induce fatigue – it is essential to get a re-test before advancing the programme up a notch.

There are two classic syndromes which are associated with rapid fatigue and breathlessness.

1. *Hypoglycaemia* – this comes about by an abnormally low sugar level in the blood. Although quite rare, there have been three cases recorded during the executive programme the authors have been associated with.

One example was quite serious – the reconstruction of the event is as follows:

An executive left for work at 4.30am on a Monday morning after a weekend in the country, driving for two and a half hours to reach the gymnasium by seven in the morning. Note: he had no breakfast or even a drink before leaving home. He had a fairly active work-out, including 35 minutes running on the treadmill at 7.5 miles per hour, 10 kilometres on the static cycle, and a circuit on the multigym. This circuit was followed by a ten minute sauna and shower. The executive got to his desk by 9 o'clock and sat in meetings through until 4.30pm, during the whole time he only drank black coffee without sugar. At this time he felt sick and nauseous, cleared up his paper work and set off home in the London traffic around 5 o'clock.

Driving along a main London road in dense traffic he began to perspire profusely and fainted at the wheel of his car, going at 50 m.p.h. and accelerating. He was taken from the wrecked car by ambulance to hospital. There was no evidence of damage apart from minor abrasions. The tests that followed ten to fifteen minutes later indicated that his blood pressure was normal 116/78, and that his pulse (electro cardiogram) was stable and regular at fifty-two beats per minute.

The doctors were concerned about the apparent low pulse rate until it was explained that he regularly worked out and that that was his normal pulse rate, at rest. It is a point to be borne in mind that you should communicate this to your doctor for reference purposes!

The initial diagnosis was either:–

- Food poisoning
- Stomach upset (gastro enteritis)
- Low sugar level in the blood (hypoglycaemia)

On reconstructing the day's events it was agreed that hypoglycaemia was the cause.

To avoid future occurrences a specialist advised breakfast daily with a cup of tea with sugar (not coffee), cut down on coffee intake, and have balanced regular meals through the day. Proceed with normal work routine and exercise programme as though nothing had happened. The executive has had no recurrence of the syndrome since that happened. There have been two other recorded incidents, but not so severe.

This is yet another case of knowing your own metabolism and ensuring that you take time out on a regular basis to have a balanced lifestyle.

2. *Hyperventilation* – In this particular syndrome, anxiety builds up concern about breathing and rapidly develops into a feeling of inability to get enough air into the lungs. The feeling of being out-of-breath accentuates over-breathing and results in lowering the CO_2 level in the blood – this is present in air being exhaled. The results of this gives sensations of numbness, tingling at the body extremities and light headedness. The syndrome is normally associated with nervous and tense persons – please refer to cautionary observations page 36.

Aches and Pains

Pain is the result of pressure, irritation, or disruption of nerve endings situated throughout the body. One's tolerance of pain appears to be dependent upon hereditary factors, general personality, motivation influences, and the extent or severity of trauma.

The obscure aches and pains that many experience (especially in later life) are often due to occupational stresses and habitual bad posture.

Executives, in particular, may find themselves more predisposed to postural aches and pains, due to extended periods in a car or plane, at the desk or at meetings. More recent are the hazards of using the keyboard of the terminal, viewing the visual display unit, and constantly working in artificial light with little or no regard to ergonomics.

The long term results of working in these conditions may lead to adaptive shortening of ligaments and muscles with localised muscle fatigue and associated arthritic conditions. Specific aches and pains are often located in the regions of the neck, across the shoulders and the lower back. Ultimately, postural problems become chronic and may need specific and specialised attention.

Extended periods of sitting at a desk, at meetings, lunching, or when travelling, set up strains in the anti-gravity muscles of the neck and back which ultimately give way to the ever-present gravitational forces. The shoulders and head tend to drop forward and the body adopts a slumped position unless there is a counter-balance.

The pressures exerted may result in acute pain between the shoulder blades and lower back which, unless corrected, may become chronic. Each individual has characteristics that affect posture. To avoid these aches and pains, it is necessary to ensure that balance, stability and the neutralisation of the effects of gravity are effected through the most economic muscular activity. Other aches and pains may be due to badly designed furniture, car seats and bed mattresses; it is worthwhile to examine the application of ergonomics.

Desks and tables should be adjusted to suit the height of the individual using them, so that 'slumping' is minimised. Chairs should also be at a height that allows the feet to reach the floor comfortably, and with a firm back which should, as much as possible, fit the natural contours of the spine. The best mattresses are those that offer firm support evenly over their entire area, rather than those that are too easily affected by forces of weight distribution. Pillows too, should be comfortable but firm, not holding the head too high nor too low. The odd aches that one sometimes experiences on getting out of bed in the mornings are usually due to joint stiffness and will generally ease off within a short time of attending to the daily routine.

There are, of course, the aches and pains of unaccustomed work, that we all experience following a day's gardening or during a holiday when we tend to become more physically active. These are perhaps reminders that one should maintain a reasonable level of fitness throughout one's life.

One thing is certain, aches and pains are the body's response to trauma. Mostly the trauma is of a not very serious nature, but it should never be completely ignored. When in doubt consult a physician, if only to eliminate more sinister causes. A lifestyle may predispose one towards certain acceptable aches and pains, but many of these can be largely eliminated by regular exercise.

Lack of Flexibility

Perhaps one of the most recognisable symptoms arising out of long term physical inactivity is a progressive deterioration of joint mobility and muscle extensibility. This is largely due to the adaptive shortening of connective tissue which gradually takes place in individuals leading sedentary lifestyles.For some persons there may exist a selective impairment of flexibility affecting only certain joints. This may be due to inherent characteristics that cannot easily be rectified.

One should also be aware that one's body type will tend to affect the degree of flexibility in certain areas. However, it is certain that the regular performance of the right type of exercise will improve one's general degree of flexibility.

It is important to understand that exercises (performed at speed), involving extreme ranges of joint movement, will activate a projective reflex which will inhibit, rather than improve flexibility. Therefore, jerky or bouncy movements are not recommended, indeed in some instances they may cause serious joint and muscle injury. Reference to the explanations accompanying illustrations of the flexibility exercises in this book will indicate that the best method is by the use of 'static stretch' whereby the muscles are put to their greatest length and held for a period.

The desirable degree of flexibility will differ according to the aspirations of the individual. Those who endeavour to excel in some form of sport or game will want to attain as supple a body as possible. Even those who are only concerned with general day-to-day fitness need to maintain general joint mobility. This is necessary for even simple activities like walking or running, if grace and co-ordination are to be preserved and injury avoided.

A simple rule for the maintenance of flexibility is to put all joints through a full range of movement at least three times per week.

II

Fitness Assessment – A Ready Reckoner

Although there are many tests of fitness, the following four categories suffice for a fitness 'yardstick'.

1. Pulse recovery rate.
2. Power tests which include abdominal, upper and lower limbs.
3. Flexibility of the shoulders, lateral and forward spinal flexion and the hips.
4. Ideal weight and body composition.

These tests enable anyone, from the very unfit to the very fit, to assess their own fitness level.

The tests should be undertaken before commencing the training programme. Adjustments can be made to the work schedule if the tests are carried out at periodic intervals, say weekly, to further improve performance. Some individuals may need to modify the exercises to suit their level of ability. Modifications are explained and illustrated later in this book.

1. The pulse recovery rate – tests general cardio vascular fitness. It involves measuring the pulse recovery rate following a period of activity that makes demands on the blood transport system, and can be performed by both men and women of any age group – in the absence of ill health it is perfectly safe.

The person undertaking this test should:

- Not eat for two hours prior to the test, and
- Rest for five minutes prior to the test

Using a bench, chair, stool or step at least 12 inches high – step up and down to a count of four, i.e. (1) left foot up, (2) right foot up (3) left foot down (4) right foot down, and so on, finishing with both feet on the ground. The rate should be approximately two complete step-ups every five seconds. The test is completed after 72 step-ups which will last some 3 minutes. Sit down and check the pulse rate for ten seconds then multiply by six to get Beats Per Minute.

Here is the ready reckoner, ranging from poor to excellent within each age group.

Pulse Rate 1 Minute After Test

Classification	*Age 20–39*	*Age 40–55*	*Age 56–65*
Excellent	71– 78	76– 83	79– 86
Very Good	79– 83	84– 88	87– 91
Average	84– 99	89–104	92–107
Below Average	100–107	105–115	108–118
Poor	108–118	116–126	119–130

TABLE 2

Note: When taking the pulse – place three fingers over the radial artery located on the thumb side of the wrist, or on the neck just below the angle of the jaw.

2. Power tests (see over) – these provide a series of strength measurements. It is important that before undertaking these tests some warm-up pre-stretch exercises are completed to avoid injury see p.44. Do not push yourself to extremes unless you are a trained athlete.

Test 1 Sit-Ups (abdominal muscle power) *Figs 33/34*

To Be Completed in 30 Seconds (½ Minute)

Classification	*Age 20–39*	*Age 40–55*	*Age 56–65*
Excellent	18+	15+	10+
Very Good	12–17	10–14	6–9
Average	7–11	5–9	3–5
Below Average	3–6	2–4	1–2
Poor	Below 3	Below 2	None

TABLE 3

Test 2 Press-Ups (upper limbs power) *Figs 39/40*

To Be Completed in 30 Seconds (½ Minute)

Classification	*Age 20–39*	*Age 40–55*	*Age 56–65*
Excellent	25+	20+	15+
Very Good	18–24	14–19	10–14
Average	10–17	8–13	5–8
Below Average	4–9	3–7	2–4
Poor	Below 4	Below 3	Below 2

TABLE 4

Test 3 Single Leg Squat (lower limbs power) *Fig 29*

To Be Completed in 30 Seconds (½ Minute)

Classification	*Age 20–39*	*Age 40–55*	*Age 56–65*
Excellent	18+	15+	12+
Very Good	15–17	12–14	8–11
Average	12–14	8–11	5–7
Below Average	8–11	5–7	2–4
Poor	Below 8	Below 5	Below 2

Note: Each leg to be tested separately

TABLE 5

3. Flexibility – this series tests the flexibility of the shoulders, lateral and forward flexion of the spine and mobility of the hips. These tests are not related to age or sex.

Forward spinal flexion: Sit on the floor with legs outstretched then reach forward as far as possible with both hands. The finger tips should reach at least to the ankles without bending the knees.

FIGURE 1

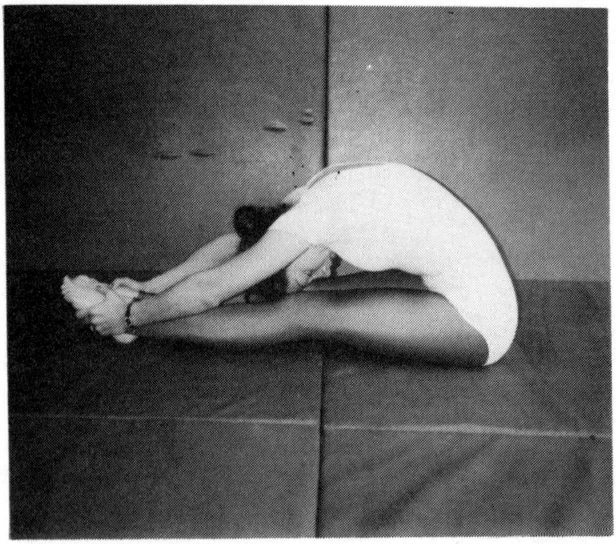

Lateral spine flexion: Stand with the feet approximately 24″ apart keeping the shoulders erect – reach down first to the right and then to the left as far as possible. The finger tips should reach to mid calf.

FIGURE 2

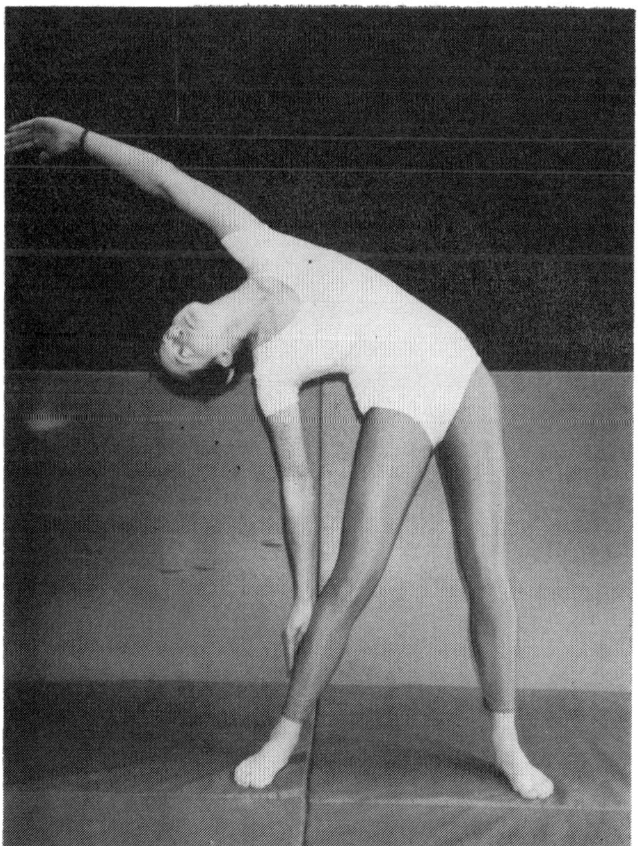

Shoulder flexibility: should enable both arms to be raised above the head with elbows straight. The upper arms should be adjacent to the ears without lowering the head.

FIGURE 3

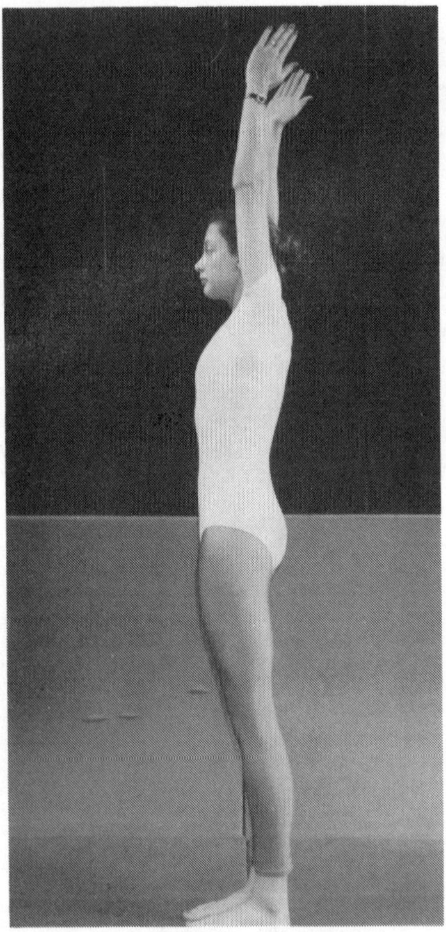

Flexibility of the hips: Stand – raise one leg sideways onto a stool, bench, chair or stair, at least 12″ high. Keeping the shoulders well back reach down the side of the raised leg. The finger tips should reach at least to mid calf.

FIGURE 4

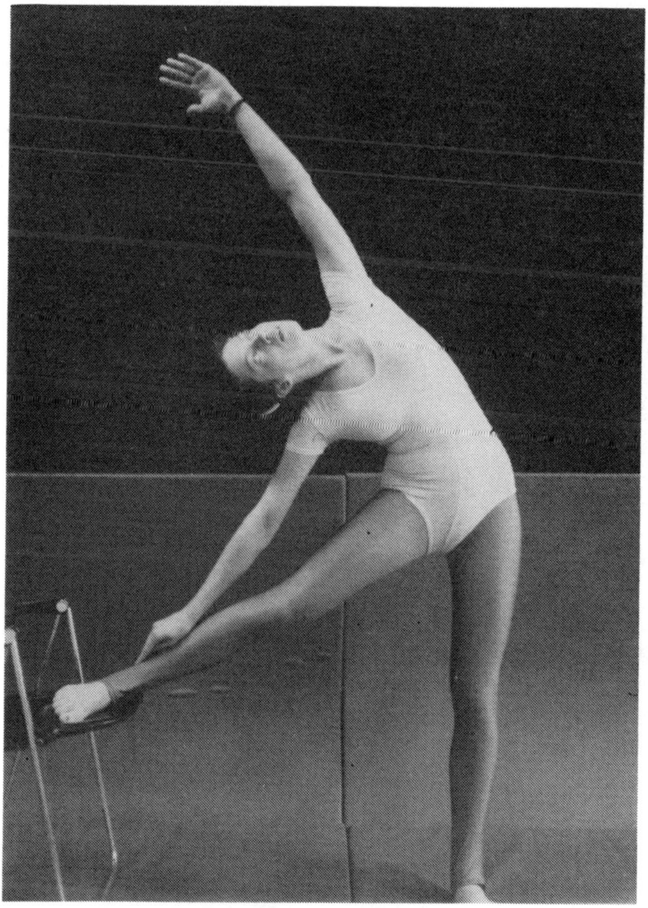

Sitting on the floor with the foot of one leg held over the thigh of the straight leg. Exert gentle pressure with the elbow pressing the bent knee downwards. Hold for 10 seconds, repeat with each leg 3 times.

FIGURE 5

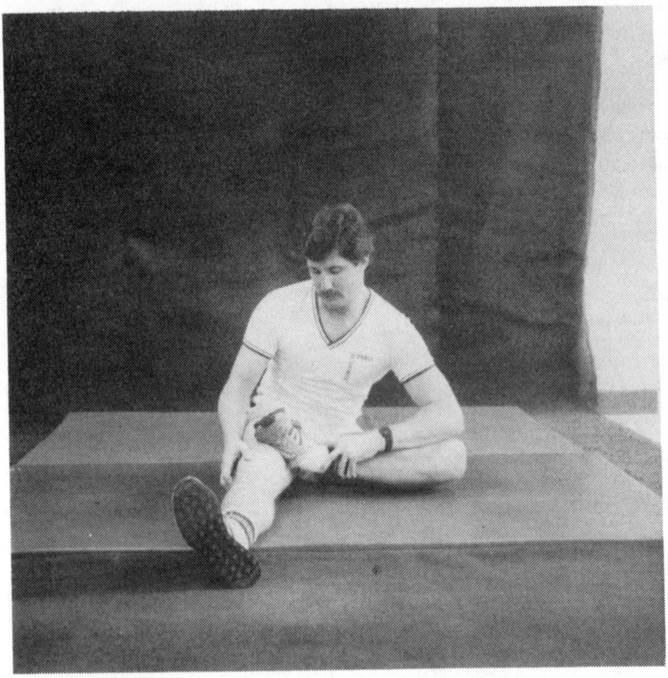

4. Ideal weight and body composition – these tests have been purposely left until last – when the dreaded result of over indulgence is most readily revealed. The tests seek to determine the ideal weight and body composition.

   - The pinch test – allow your arm to hang, pinch the area on the underside of the arm between the shoulder and elbow pulling the skin away from the underlying muscle.
     If the fold of skin is more than ½″ you are too fat and need a weight control programme.

   - The ideal weight test – multiply every inch in excess of five feet by six then add 106 lbs (male). For women, multiply every inch over five feet by five then add 100 lbs.

   For example:

Man						
HEIGHT	5′10″	=	10×6	=	60
	60	+	106	=	166 lbs ideal weight
Woman						
HEIGHT	5′3″	=	3×5	=	15
	15	+	100	=	115 lbs ideal weight

TABLE 6

This gives a close approximation to height/weight relationship.
Refer for further details to chapters on obesity and weight control.

III

How To Proceed

If you can identify with, and relate to, the problems outlined and you decide that your fitness level is not up to standard, you may decide to proceed or stop right there. The temptation to rectify the problem is normally overwhelming and if you decide to proceed then you should, at the outset, decide to follow at least a three month programme to enable you to measure the impact it has had on you.

The exciting thing is that you will see immediate results and your only challenge will be to improve against your previous efforts. Naturally, there will be lapses for all sorts of reasons, but having discovered that you *can* achieve an improvement, however small, you will be greatly encouraged.

It is extremely important that, within all the limits set by age, body type, fitness at the outset and so on, you establish a positive attitude and that you totally agree with the programme, as then you will feel committed to yourself (not someone else). If your mind accepts the 'challenge' your body will never let you down – apart from injury.

First, it is essential to have a comprehensive health screening.

Second, ensure you invest time and effort getting the correct apparel. Note: excellent shoes are essential – refer equipment portfolio, Appendix 3.

Third, always complete what you set out to accomplish. (Never cheat on yourself.)

Fourth, establish a regular routine, including stretch exercises before and after a work out.

Fifth, do not diet without exercise – do not lose weight too rapidly but establish a balanced approach.

Sixth, ensure you get adequate rest and relaxation.

Seventh, do not be too ambitious – one step at a time. Upgrade your programme only under supervision.

EXERCISE REGULARLY – GO AT IT SLOWLY

DON'T EAT AND DRINK EXCESSIVELY!!

Motivation

What is the spur that starts people thinking about a fitness programme, why do they continue, why do they drop out?

Initial interest can range from chance remarks by family, friends or colleagues about size, new suits, extra collar size, to a personal awareness of deterioration in fitness level. Whatever source the initial interest stems from, the awareness generates sufficient motivation to do something about it.

Although there are a number of key features which impel a person into participating in the programme, it would be naive to think that there were not also some negative aspects.

A high degree of motivation can be generated at the outset of the programme. The professional supervisor should do a great deal of pre-planning to ensure that the person is well prepared and the mental attitude correct.

Preparing the ground:

- Does the person suffer from stress, obesity, high blood pressure, high pulse rate and does he really want to do something to rectify these problems?
- Can he recall his fitness level at, say, 21 and does he believe he can get to that level of fitness again? Case studying and discussion will convince him it can be done.
- Will the person participating be keen enough to aim at 'par' for the course and stick with a lifelong fitness programme. That is, what will he/she do at the 'CROSSROADS' – what road will be taken?

Before taking up the programme, assess yourself against these points.

FOR	AGAINST
• Tackling known problems	• Cannot find the time
• Extended life expectancy	• Boredom with repetitive tasks
• Reduced illness incidence	• Failure to achieve goals
• Involvement	• Too many temptations
• General feeling of well-being	• Onerous work and travel schedule
• All round moderation	• Dislike of exercise
• Better equipped for favourite recreation	• Feel fit enough

Although each of the above pros and cons are not of equal weight you could give a rough assessment of how you would score (say on a scale of 1–10 for each point).

Individual (self) motivation:
Some people prefer to go it alone in an attempt to improve against their own personal best performance. There are some very dedicated people on the programme, in which the authors participate, who are motivated by their individual competition against themselves.

Group motivation:
Some people find self motivation extremely difficult. In these circumstances a group will emerge who begin to compete. Naturally, the professional supervisor can have a 'catalytic' role in developing a competitive theme. Superstars, best performance within an age group, decathlon type approach, are interesting, but should be supervised so as not to provoke injury by overdoing things. The results of such approaches are generally very rewarding not only in terms of improved fitness but also in healthy competition and camaraderie.

Cautionary Observations

The points on how to proceed are mind 'joggers'. There are some important cautionary steps that one must take if the fitness programme is to be both a pleasurable and successful experience.

1. Self analysis and observation can do much more than any doctor to maintain general fitness and well-being. People do not require expert advice to know that alcohol gradually destroys the stomach lining and attacks the liver, or that the risk of

lung disease is less if you do not smoke, or that obesity will have attendant health problems rarely experienced by the 'greyhound' breed.

Some of the more important observations that can be made during the programme are:

- Pulse rate: Regularly check your pulse rate at rest and after exercising. The test for the pulse rate at rest is best measured on waking up first thing in the morning. After exercising, means on completion of your pre-planned fitness programme. Count the number of beats in ten seconds and then multiply by six for Beats Per Minute. Any significant irregularity should be observed and accurately recorded for explanation to your doctor. Is there any irregularity such as palpitation or skipping a beat?
  Palpitation is normally associated with a high level of activity or some emotional experience, e.g. fright, causing the heart to thump.
- Weight: Fluctuations in weight are very important to observe and monitor. Keep a regular log and know what your ideal weight should be.
- Temperature: Every household should have a 'thermometer' and every member of the household should know how to record the exact temperature of anyone. Although you feel hot, do you in fact have a temperature?
- Body knowledge: Everyone should have a complete understanding of their body and any ache, pain, irregularity or change can be observed and recorded.

2. Skin Fungus: It is quite common when working out and showering in communal areas to contract

forms of skin fungus. Fungal infections of the skin are not serious and will normally be rectified by regular cleaning, drying and powder application to keep the affected area dry.

The most common skin fungal infections are athletes foot and 'jock-itch'. You should never be without a proprietary brand of powder or zinc undecylenate cream.

3. Sunburn: This is one area in which you can really be a master of your own destiny. It generally results from too much time in the sun to get maximum exposure on a short trip, falling asleep, participating in outdoor sports, or drinks around the pool. It is only when blistering occurs a day or so after exposure that treatment may be needed for second degree burns. Baking soda in a bath of water (four tablespoons) is as good and as soothing as most remedies. There are many proprietary brands of protection against sunburn. Naturally, as with all the excesses, moderation is the best course of action.

4. Strains and Sprains: During the fitness programme it is probable that some minor injury will occur, unless you are extremely fortunate. Some of the more common arise from fast jerky actions, twists or turns, or a sharp blow on a particular joint such as the ankle or knee.

   You will be exposed to some of these by running on uneven surfaces (watch the pavement!) swerving for the dog when out running, letting the stool or chair you step-up on fall on the foot, some tired colleague accidentally bumping into you. You will never cease to be amazed at the novel way in which strains and sprains can be inflicted.

Ligaments may be:

- Stretched
- Partially torn
- Completely torn

The ligaments are tissues that hold the joints in place and provide stability. Undue stress on a joint such as a turn, twist or blow can result in strains, sprains or tears.

You should know your body and any indication of pain means that you should rest. It is a fallacy to think you can run or exercise out of pain (only stiffness).

If you have pain or swelling apply a cold water compress, or ice-cubes in a towel to the painful area to arrest any internal bleeding or further damage. After you have applied the cold compress, support with the aid of an elastic bandage until the swelling goes down and the pain subsides – rest is essential. If there is no relief from pain or sleeplessness within 48 hours seek expert advice.

5. Stomach problems: The executive suffers more than most from stomach problems. Heavy travel schedules to far away exotic places take their toll on the anatomy:

   - Ice cold beer
   - New local dishes to try
   - Local water (BEWARE ice in your drink)
   - Seafood delicacies to titillate the palate

   Some people have the constitution that defies all the temptations laid before them – others have a double share of sympathetic suffering.

6. Hyperventilation: This occurs when the CO_2 level in the blood falls as a result of over breathing (see page no. 19). By breathing into a paper bag or similar, for about fifteen to twenty minutes the CO_2 level usually returns to normal, and the symptoms subside.

   Never travel without some water purification tablets or non-absorbable antacids. Have them to travel, but also at home. More extreme forms of upset stomach may cause diarrhoea or constipation and it is essential to take precautions if these extreme conditions occur.

CHECKLIST

Useful aids if problems occur (some will)

1.	Weighing Scales	+ –	Normal Weight
2.	Thermometer	+ –	Normal Temperature 98.4°F, 36.8°C
3.	Skin Fungus		Anti-Fungal Aids
4.	Sunburn		Sunscreen Aids
5.	Sprains and Strains		Ice/Cold Water Elastic Bandages
6.	Stomach Problems Upsets Constipation Diarrhoea	 – – –	 Antacids Laxatives Kaopectate

IV

Fitness Programme

Before embarking on the fitness programme it is extremely important to understand that there is a significant difference in body types and their relationship to exercise. The differing body structures will affect the way in which varying physical activities are accomplished. Although this should be obvious, it is seldom taken into account by authorities advocating fitness training. Sometimes this can have a demoralising effect on individuals attempting to improve their fitness levels.

A training programme should consider not only age and sex but also genetic influences on body type and personality. (A tailor-made programme should be devised for each individual, taking these factors into account).

Perhaps an analogy will help:

Horses range in type from racing, pulling heavy loads, polo, trekking, etc. So individuals have inherited certain characteristics – which should predetermine the most suitable sport or training method. Pause, think and be selective!

Three distinct body types can be identified:

- Endomorphs – rotund individuals. They tend to be overweight. They are generally well suited to power sports such as wrestling, weight lifting and swimming.

- Mesomorphs – typified by their athletic build, muscular and broad shouldered. Normally associated with speed and agility.
- Ectomorphs – typically slim and linear. They excel at activities demanding endurance, often possessing good weight/power ratios. Generally associated with body-raising sports such as high, long and triple jumps.

Few people fit exactly into any one of these categories, but the dominant body type is usually apparent.

The dominant body types can influence, enhance or limit, performances in sporting activities.

Finally, it should be noted that no amount of training will affect the body types, although certain unwanted extremes can be modified.

The general fitness programme sets out to explain how to tackle specific points identified and explained in the introduction and the chapter on fitness problems. Furthermore, the programme now to be outlined explains how a person can get to grips with deviations from the 'norm' identified in the fitness assessment explained earlier.

It is important to follow the hints on how to proceed and then get stuck in if you want results.

The authors have identified the 'CARAFE' syndrome - which demonstrates that the increased activity outlined in the programme counterbalances executive lifestyle problems. To reach 'par' may only take 6–8 weeks. The following illustration demonstrates this phenomenon.

The fitness programme normally goes through five stages.

1. Total Imbalance: At this stage there is no participation in the programme and all the problems of stress, over-indulgence, high blood pressure, rapid fatigue including breathlessness, aches and pains, loss of energy and lack of flexibility are prevalent.

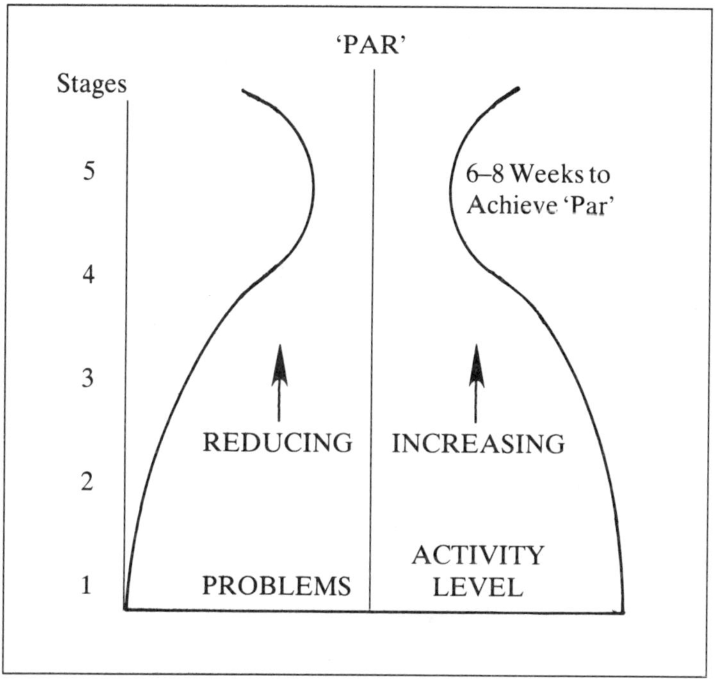

TABLE 7

2. Assessment: This stage is the exciting time of determining against the fitness 'ready reckoner' the individual level of fitness and how big a target one has to aim for to reach (or exceed) par for the course.

3. Activity: The start of pre-stretch, flexibility, aerobics and power exercises with a gradual build-up which will begin to offset many of the problems induced by the executive lifestyle.

4. 'Par': The individual achieves or exceeds 'par for the course' – the balance between problems, level of activity and diet.

5. Crossroads: Should you decide to scale greater heights of achievement? Or revert to the inactive problem – riddled lifestyle? Or just retain the balanced way of life?

Everyone tends to go through the stages and begins to question and assess the many variable factors that lead to individual balance.

Self analysis at each stage is important: competing with oneself is exciting and without doubt extremely satisfying.

The events to be tackled in the activity stage fall into five categories:

- Pre-stretch
- Flexibility
- Aerobics
- Power activities (musculo-skeletal)
- Post-stretch

You *must* start with the pre-stretch exercises and end with the post-stretch warm-down. The other three categories can be varied depending on individual preference. But it is important to complete the full programme to achieve a balance.

ALWAYS COMPLETE WHAT YOU SET OUT TO DO

Pre-Stretch Exercises

The following exercises must precede any vigorous activity. The movements must be carried out smoothly without jerking or bouncing. Each stretch position should be held for about eight seconds, and each exercise repeated at least four times.

Start your pre-stretch with gentle head circling in both directions and in as full a range as possible.

Windmill: Circle the arms backwards alternately, pushing the hands away and bringing the upper arm close to the ear. Then repeat with both arms circling together.

FIGURE 6

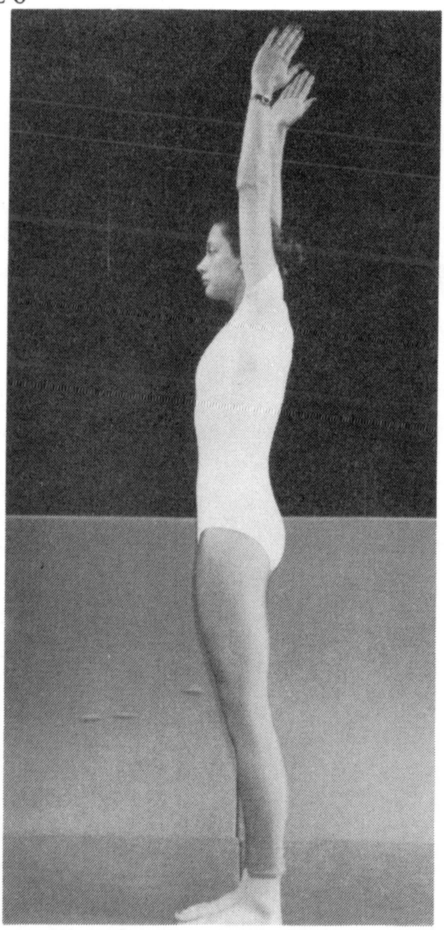

Back scratcher stretch: With one arm reach down towards the space between the shoulder blades, the other hand being placed over the elbow joint to push slowly down the back bone to the point of tension, repeat with other arm.

FIGURE 7

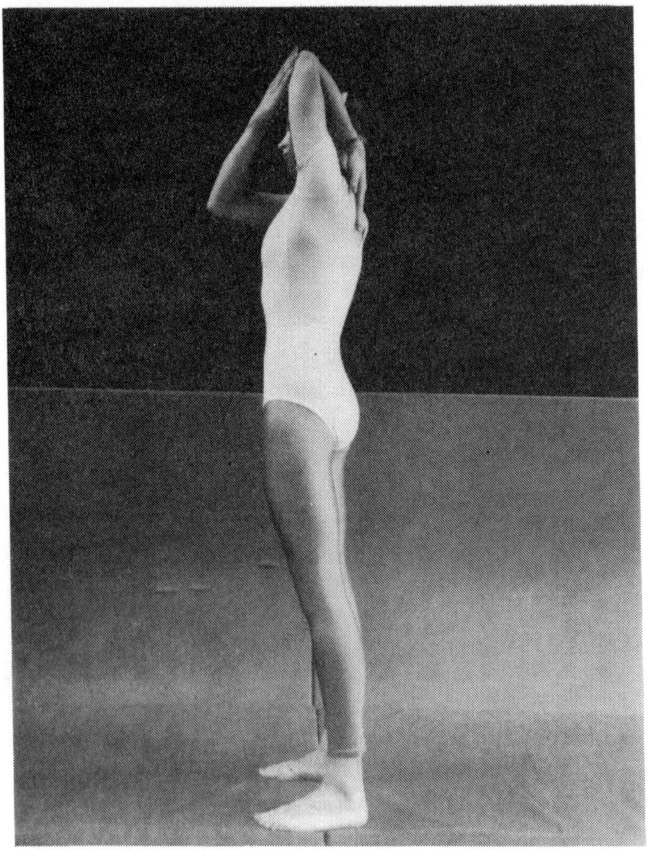

The twister: Standing feet astride, raise both elbows sideways to 90° and interlace the fingers. Keeping feet firmly anchored, rotate the trunk with elbows assisting the range of tension. Repeat other side.

FIGURE 8

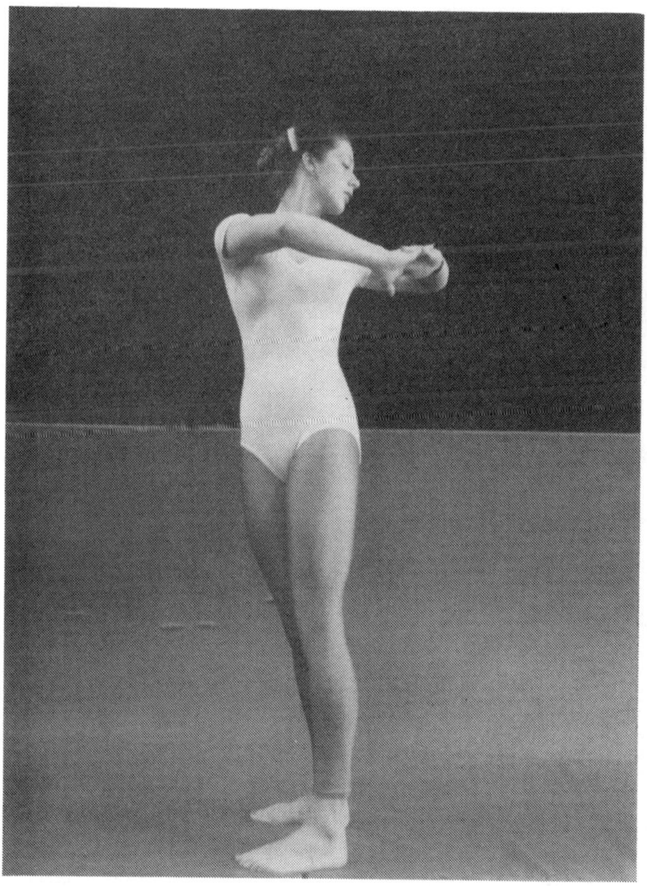

Side stretch: Stand feet astride. Keeping the shoulders pulled well back, reach as far down the side of the leg as possible as the other arm is raised and held close to the ear. Repeat each side.

FIGURE 9

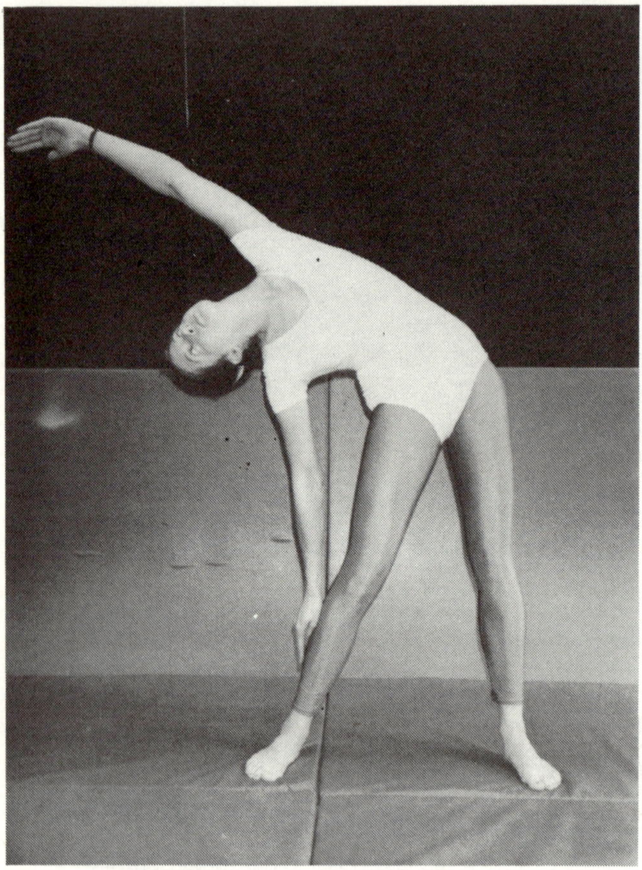

Straddle stretch: Feet astride as wide as possible, bend knees and place both hands flat on floor. Making sure that the hands do not lift, slowly try to straighten the knees as you rock the weight of the body backwards. If you succeed in straightening the knees, further stretch can be obtained by bending at the elbows.

FIGURE 10

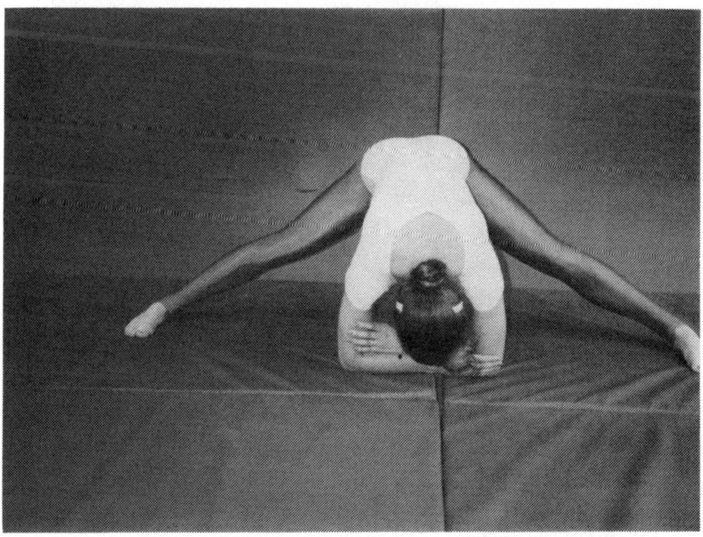

Thigh stretch: Stand with support from wall or chair-back. Bend one knee raising the foot behind, grasp the foot with the free hand and pull it upwards and backwards. Keep trunk upright throughout. Repeat each leg.

FIGURE 11

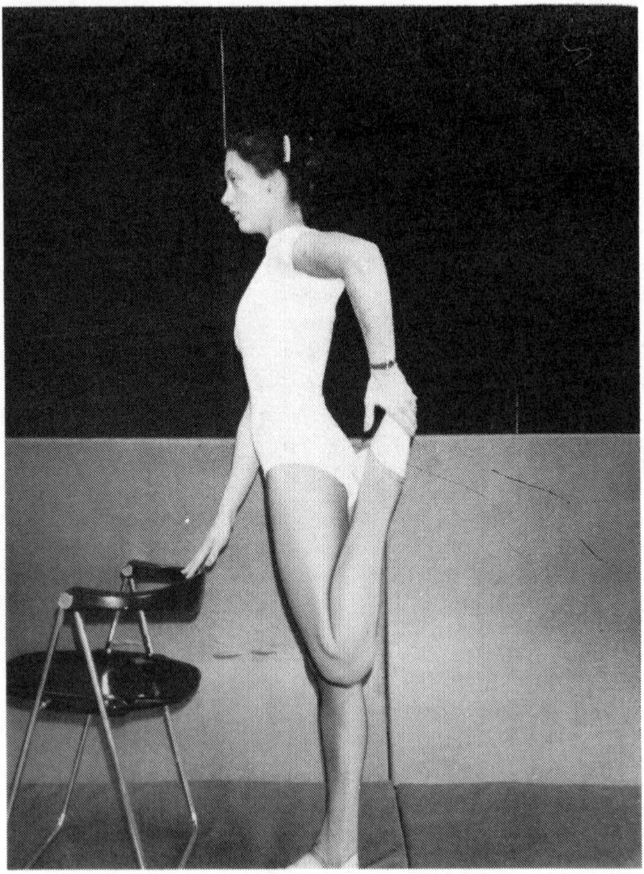

Hamstring stretch: Crouch, placing finger tips on floor, knees together. Keeping the weight of the body over the finger tips, slowly raise the hips attempting to straighten the knees. For further stretch, press chin to chest as you do the movement.

FIGURE 12

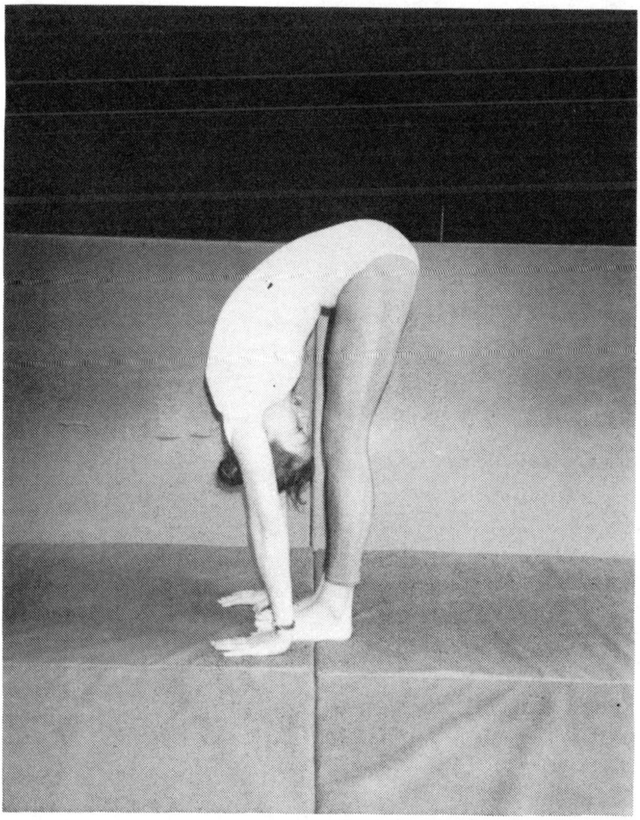

Heelcord stretch: Stand in forward lunge position with wall support. Raise toes of leading foot, with knee bent, on to a book or platform two inches high. Increase the degree of forward lunge until point of tension is reached. Repeat each leg.

FIGURE 13

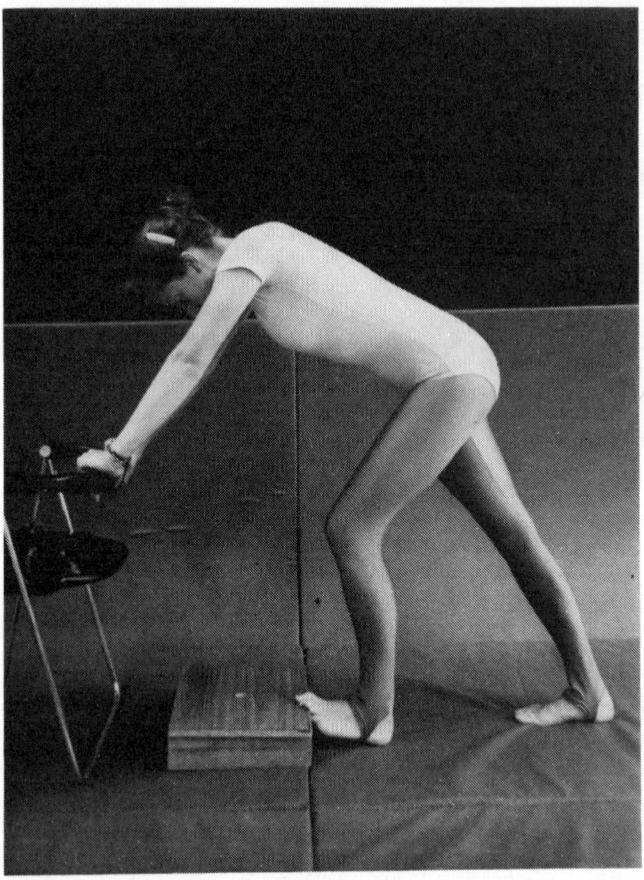

Flexibility Exercises

Perform these smoothly without jerking or bouncing. Since the pre-stretch exercises deal adequately with shoulder flexibility, this section concerns mostly the spine, hips and knees.

Start doing each exercise six times, increase by two repetitions per week until you reach twenty, at which point maintain.

Side lying leg raising: Lie on your side with lower leg bent at the knee and head resting on your forearm. Raise upper leg as high as possible.

FIGURE 14

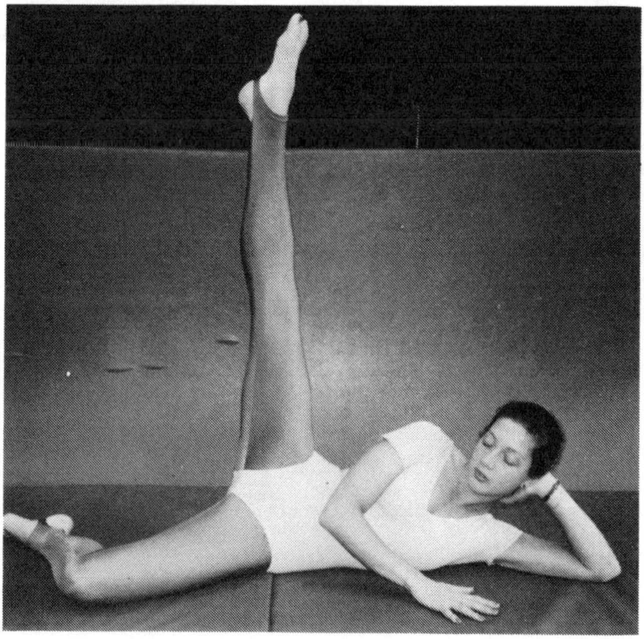

Side lying: As above, carry upper leg forwards and backwards as far as possible.

FIGURE 15

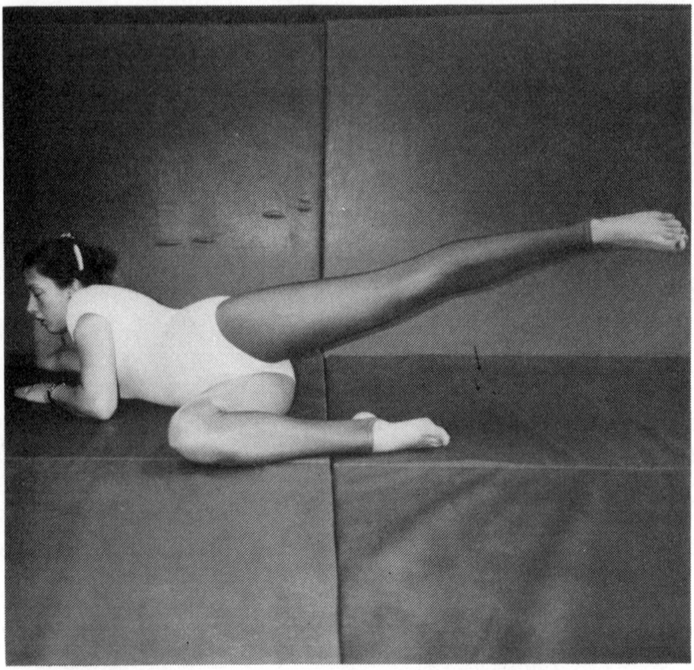

Back lying knees bent: Raise both knees onto chest and using the arms pull them up tight raising the head at the same time, then return to starting position.

FIGURE 16

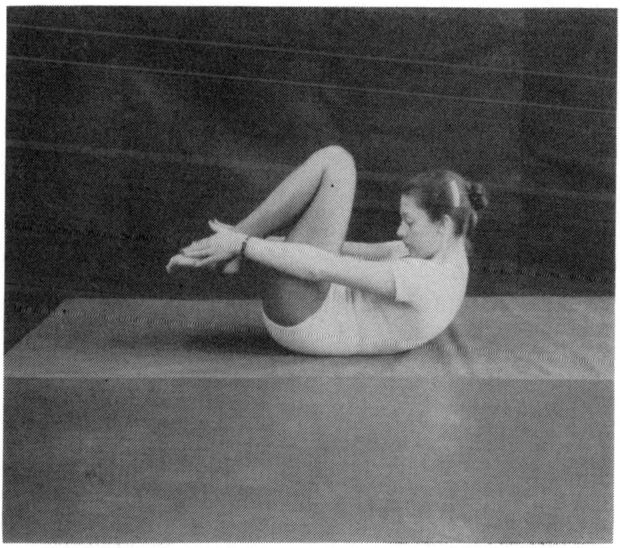

Starting position as before: raise both knees onto chest and rock backwards bringing the knees up and over your head, the hands should press down on floor at level of hips. Do not straighten the knees if discomfort is experienced.

FIGURE 17

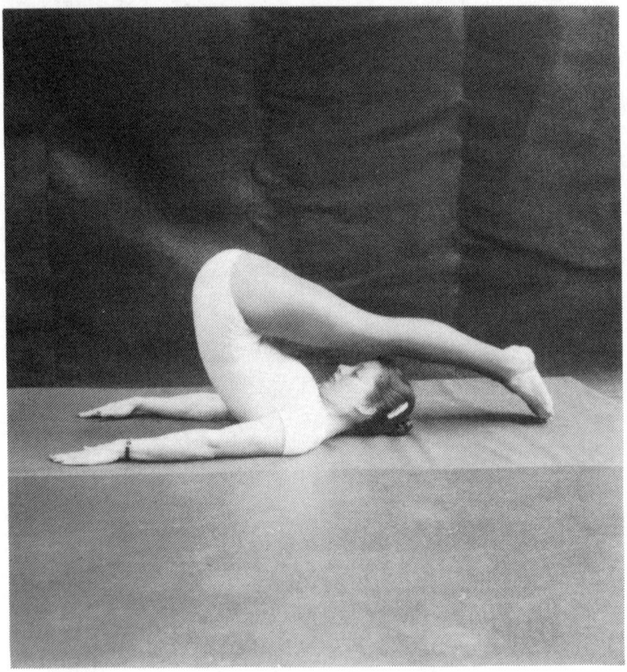

Back lying, legs straight, arms out to 90°: Bend one knee and bring it across the stomach attempting to touch opposite hand with the foot. Do not move the hands.

FIGURE 18

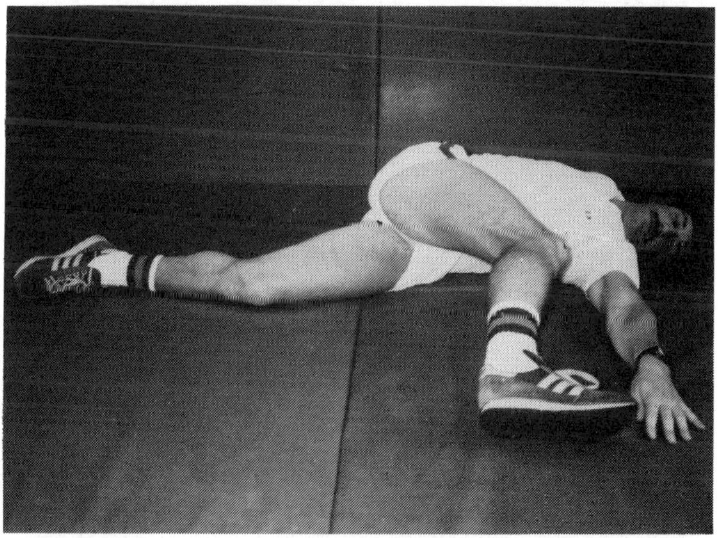

On hands and knees: With hands well in advance of the shoulders elbows straight throughout, rock forwards bringing the front of the hips down to the floor and pressing the head backwards. Then rock backwards as far as possible bringing the forehead down to the floor.

FIGURE 19

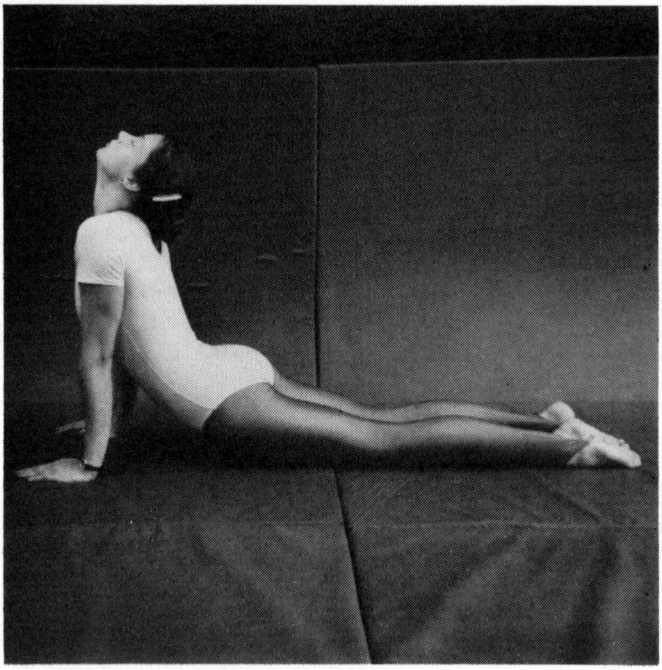

Aerobics

The ability of the human body to carry out continuous work for long periods is largely dependent upon the response to the activity by the heart, lungs and muscles.

By imposing a demand on these at regular intervals great improvements are possible in activities that call for endurance. This is because the oxygen transport system of the body will adapt to the work-loads. Thus, the heart will develop a stronger, more efficient pumping action, the lungs will increase their ventilation and exertion, and the blood vessels will gain greater vascularisation to the muscles. This type of training is known as Aerobic, which means, 'in the presence of oxygen.' In the absence of oxygen the skeletal muscles can work only for a short time due to a rapid build-up of lactic acid and limitation of energy-producing chemicals. This 'anaerobic' activity leads to an oxygen debt which is only repaid after a suitable period of recovery.

Activities of medium or low intensity can be carried out for extremely long periods of time even though there is a slow build-up of lactic acid which eventually leads to fatigue. With aerobic training, fatigue levels are delayed as endurance levels are increased.

The key to aerobic exercise efficiency is found in the ability of the cardio-vascular system to supply the cells with oxygen in sufficient quantity to meet the demand. This is known as oxygen uptake and is one of the methods by which the fitness of an individual can be measured.

In sustained effort, athletes often reach their maximum oxygen uptake and this can be closely correlated with their total output of energy. Through many areas of research in the field of exercise physiology, figures have been produced that give approximate levels of maximum oxygen uptake for given work loads. For example, in Kenneth Cooper's book 'The New Aerobics'

he states that a maximum oxygen uptake of between 42.6 ml/kg/min. and 51.5 ml/kg/min. measured in terms of a young man running a distance of 1¾ miles in 12 minutes gives a fitness category of 'good'.
ml/kg/min=Millilitres per Kilogram per Minute.
Millilitres=Oxygen. Kilogram=Weight.

Although aerobic training will improve endurance, the extent to which an individual may improve depends to a certain degree on the genetic influence, and on his body-type. Lean body-types usually do much better than stocky muscular or heavily-built individuals in endurance activity.

It is of little benefit to have a fine physique without also having an efficient cardio-vascular system. Priority should therefore be given to aerobic activity, so that the individual is ensured that the oxygen transport system is equal to the tasks imposed by the working muscles.

The important factor in the selection of the right exercise for aerobic training is that it should be such that, during its execution, it does not allow even short periods of recovery. This is not always understood by sportsmen when they are told that their chosen activity is of little value in increasing cardio-vascular endurance, even though they may find the activity exhausting.

The game of squash for example, may not have a great cardio-vascular benefit unless played for two or three hours, but steady running for 20 minutes will certainly improve endurance for squash if carried out regularly. Circulo-respiratory endurance is most evident in work of medium intensity involving the whole body.

All exercise demands certain adaptations in the circulatory and respiratory systems but, in mild exercise, necessary adjustments are hardly noticed. In exercise of great intensity, such as weight-lifting, local muscle fatigue may set in before any great demands are made upon the heart and lungs. In activities such as running, cycling, swimming and brisk walking, which involve rapid and prolonged action of many muscle groups, it is circulo-respiratory efficiency which will delay the onset of fatigue. This quality, although easily recognised, is difficult to measure satisfactorily.

The level to which an individual's heart rate rises during any exercise depends on his relative physical fitness. The poorer the fitness, the less strenuous will be the activity to raise his pulse rate to 150 beats per minute.

The person who leads a sedentary life devoid of exercise might need only to walk briskly for a few minutes, whereas a trained athelete may require a sharp run for about 10 minutes. Therefore, it is possible for a poorly conditioned person to start out with relatively light exercise and still receive a training benefit. It is of course, very important to embark upon an aerobic exercise programme at a level consistent with one's age, sex, and general physical condition. Only harm can come to an untrained person starting out too fast, too far, too soon. It is wrong for any person, however qualified, to suggest levels of activity for individuals without knowing them well, but as a general guide to the rate of progression, the indices set out below indicate a possible safe exercise increase based upon heart-rate response. The *beginner* however, should always bear in mind that exercise should not be 'suffered' and, if activities of any kind become more than a pleasant exertion, the individual should ease off, even if his suggested heart-rate has not been reached.

Taking the pulse – place three fingers over the radial artery located on the thumb side of the wrist. You will then feel the pulsations as the heart pumps. This

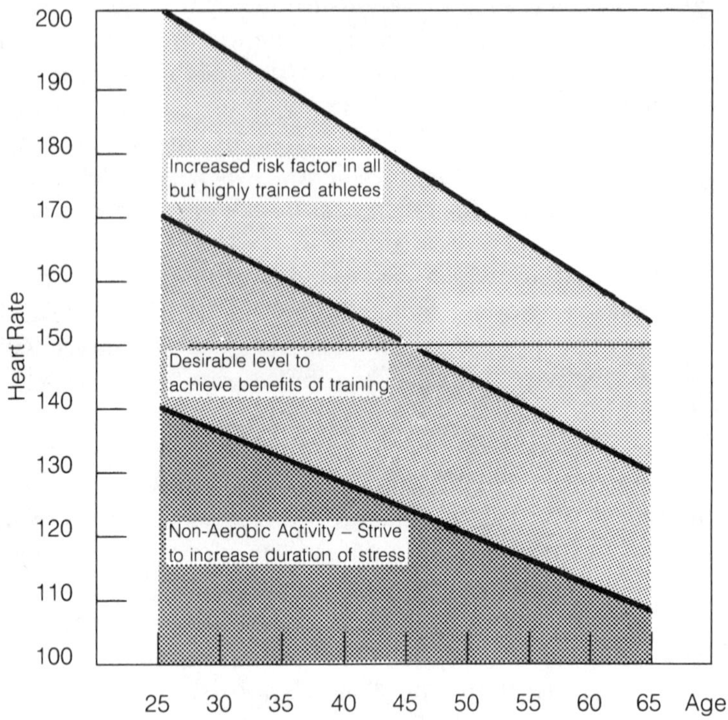

TABLE 8

should be done immediately after cessation of exercise, as the rate drops rapidly when activity stops. Count the pulse only for the first ten seconds then multiply by six. It is difficult for a complete beginner to assess how much exercise he should start with and, short of stopping to count his pulse every minute or so (which would largely defeat the object of the exercise) he must experiment until he finds his level. The index below has been researched with 150 beginners of age groups between twenty and sixty plus and represents the level at which the average participant reached his

JOGGING INDEX

Week	*20–30*	*30–40*	*40–45*	*45–50*	*50–55*	*55–60*	*60–65*
1	6 mph 5 mins	5 mph 5 mins	5 mph 5 mins	4.5 mph 5 mins	4 mph 5 mins	3.5 mph 5 mins	3.5 mph 5 mins
2	6 mph 7 mins	6 mph 5 mins	6 mph 5 mins	5.5 mph 5 mins	4.5 mph 5 mins	4 mph 5 mins	4 mph 5 mins
3	6 mph 10 mins	6 mph 7 mins	6 mph 7 mins	6 mph 5 mins	5.5 mph 5 mins	4.5 mph 5 mins	4.5 mph 5 mins
4	1¼ miles	6 mph 10 mins	6 mph 9 mins	6 mph 7 mins	6 mph 5 mins	5.5 mph 5 mins	5 mph 5 mins
5	1½ miles	1¼ miles	6 mph 10 mins	6 mph 9 mins	6 mph 7 mins	6 mph 5 mins	5.5 mph 5 mins
6	7.5 mph 12 mins	7.5 mph 12 mins	1¼ miles	1 mile	6 mph 8 mins	6 mph 7 mins	6 mph 5.5 mins

Progress by moving to a lower age category for each succeeding week.

TABLE 9

In some cases progression may be achieved more rapidly than indicated, but post exercise pulse rates should be checked to determine that they fall within the safe levels.

heart rate range of benefit through jogging over a period of six weeks at thrice-weekly training stints. Running speed can be adjudged very closely by accepting that the speed at which one is forced to break into a jog is about 5.75 mph.

It will be seen by this index (Table 9) that a run of 7.5 mph for 12 minutes is considered sufficient for the maintenance of a reasonably fit level, it bears repeating that there should be at least three work-outs a week.

There is no reason why an individual should not progress beyond the final stage on the index, but it must be said that the accumulated benefit does not necessarily equate with the extra output of effort. For those who prefer cycling and have purchased a suitable static exercise bicycle (referred to in the equipment portfolio), the index indicates (Table 10) approximate stages of progression.

Other forms of aerobic exercise are listed in Table 11 with the performance comparisons.

It will be found that some may be able to progress at a faster rate than is indicated. Table 10 is intended as a guideline to ensure safe levels of progression, particularly in the older age brackets.

Post exercise pulse rates should be checked to determine that they fall within the recommendations set out on page 62, before progression is sanctioned.

Whatever type of activity you choose for aerobic training, or whether you vary your programme, using several means to improve endurance levels, one thing is certain, provided the work-outs become a regular pattern of life, the benefits gained will cover a wide range of activity. Cardio-vascular endurance is the hub of fitness.

STATIC CYCLE FITNESS INDEX

Week	Age	20–30	30–40	40–45	45–50	50–55	55–60
1	Distance	3.2 kms	3.2 kms	3.2 kms	3.2 kms	3.2 kms	3.2 kms
	Time	10.00 m	10.30 m	10.45 m	11,00 m	11.15 m	11.30 m
	Speed	19.2 kph	18.3 kph	17.9 kph	17.5 kph	17.1 kph	17.1 kph
2	Distance	3.2 kms	3.2 kms	3.2 kms	3.2 kms	3.2 kms	3.2 kms
	Time	9.00 m	9.30 m	9.45 m	10.00 m	10.30 m	10.45 m
	Speed	21.3 kph	20.2 kph	19.7 kph	19.2 kph	18.3 kph	17.9 kph
3	Distance	3.2 kms	3.2 kms	3.2 kms	3.2 kms	3.2 kms	3.2 kms
	Time	7.45 m	8.30 m	8.45 m	9.00 m	9.30 m	9.45 m
	Speed	25.6 kph	22.6 kph	21.9 kph	21.3 kph	20.2 kph	19.7 kph
4	Distance	4.8 kms	4.8 kms	4.8 kms	4.8 kms	4.8 kms	4.8 kms
	Time	11.45 m	12.30 m	13.15 m	14.00 m	15.00 m	16.00 m
	Speed	24.5 kph	23.0 kph	21.7 kph	20.6 kph	19.2 kph	18.0 kph
5	Distance	6.4 kms	4.8 kms	4.8 kms	4.8 kms	4.8 kms	4.8 kms
	Time	15.00 m	11.45 m	12.30 m	13.15 m	14.30 m	15.30 m
	Speed	25.6 kph	24.5 kph	23.0 kph	21.7 kph	19.9 kph	18.6 kph
6	Distance	6.4 kms	6.4 kms	4.8 kms	4.8 kms	4.8 kms	4.8 kms
	Time	13.45 m	15.00 m	11.30 m	12.30 m	14.00 m	15.00 m
	Speed	28.0 kph	25.6 kph	25.0 kph	23.0 kph	20.6 kph	19.2 kph

Progress by moving to a lower age category for each succeeding week

*3.2 kms = 2 miles, 4.8 kms = 3 miles, 6.4 kms = 4 miles.

The performances for week 6 equals Fitness Category Good.

TABLE 10

ACTIVITY COMPARISON

Tennis/Squash	Walking	Swimming	Stationary Running (40–70 skips/min.)	Running	Cycling	Calories Expended
1. 10 min.	1.0ml./20-14 min.	200yds/6-5 min.	350-400 steps in 5 min.	1.0ml./20-14 min.	2ml./12-8 min.	100-120 approx.
2. 20 min.	1.5m1./22-18 min.	200yds/3 min.	800-900 steps in 10 min.	1.0ml./12-10 min.	2ml./6 min.	130
3. 30 min.	2.0m1./29-24 min.	500yds/12-8min.	900-1500 steps in 15 min.	1.0ml/10-8 min.	4m1./16-12 min.	150
4. 35 min.	2.5ml./36-30 min.	400yds/6.40 min.	1200-1400 steps in 20 min.	1.0ml./6-8 min.	5ml./20-15 min.	150+
5. 40 min.	3.0ml./43-36 min.	500yds./8 min.	1200-1350 steps in 15 min.	1.5ml./15-12 min.	6m1./24-18 min.	150-180
			(80-90 steps/min.)			
6. 45 min.	4.0ml./50-48 min.	600yds/10 min.	1400-1575 steps in 15 min.	1.5ml./12-10 min.	5m1. under 15 min.	100-200
7. 55 min.	4.0m1./80-58 min.	700yds/12 min.	1600-1800 steps in 20 min.	2.0ml/20-16 min.	8ml./32-24 min.	200-250
8. 60 min.	5.0ml./72-60 min.	800yds/13 min.		2.5ml./25-20 min.	10ml./40-30 min.	250-300
9. 80 min.		1,000 yds/17 min.		2.5ml/20-16 min.	8ml./24 min.	300-500
10. 90 min.				3.0ml./24-19 min.	10ml./30 min.	400-500+

Example: if you play 35 minutes of squash, it is equivalent to doing 2½ miles of walking in approximately 30-36 minutes, 400 yards of swimming in under 6 minutes, 20 minutes of running in place, 1 mile of running in 6-7 minutes and 5 miles of cycling in 15-19 minutes.

TABLE 11

Power Exercises (Musculo Skeletal)

The maintenance of muscle tone is quite efficiently guaranteed by regular exercise using the resistance provided by one's body weight (Isotonic), or by static contraction of muscle groups by using an immovable resistance, (Isometric).

One of the disadvantages of the latter method is that it does little to maintain muscle *endurance.* Its virtue is in its simplicity, its lack of the need for space or specialised place. In listing the following exercises, both isotonic and isometric muscle work is given for each of the principle muscle groups involved.

(Opposite) **Squat Jumps –** Calf and Thigh.
(Isotonic)
From the squat position, knees bent to 90° hands on hips. Perform a series of jumps on the spot. To intensify the exercise, try doing the jumps on and off a low bench or bottom stair tread.
DO NOT ALLOW THE KNEES TO BEND MORE THAN 90°.
(Isometric). The thigh muscles can be strongly contracted with the knee joint locked in extension. This is best done by pressing the knee backwards as the forefoot is pulled upwards. The contraction should be sustained for at least 5 seconds, then after a relaxation period, repeated. The definition of the large muscle bulk above the knee will become more pronounced if the exercise is correctly performed.

FIGURE 20

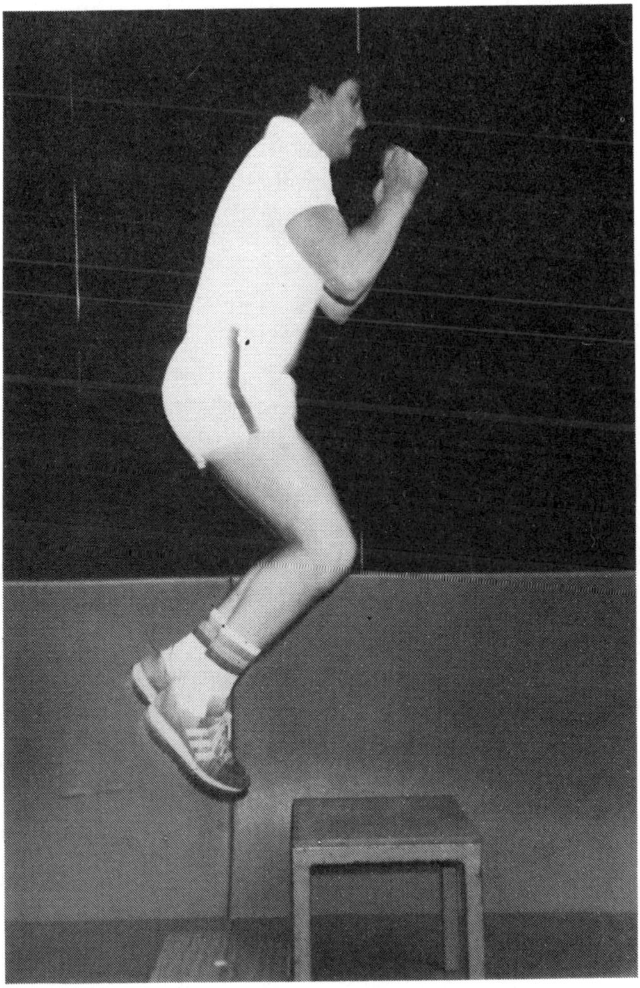

Heave Hang Pull-Ups – Upper Back, Flexors of Elbows. (Isotonic).
Some door frames are sturdy enough to provide support for this exercise. Lower support can be utilised by starting the pull-up from a 'heave hanging' position, the heels resting on the floor. (Isometric). By linking the fingers of each hand above the head, a downwards pull is exerted upon the top of the crown. Each pull should be sustained for approximately ten seconds.

FIGURE 21

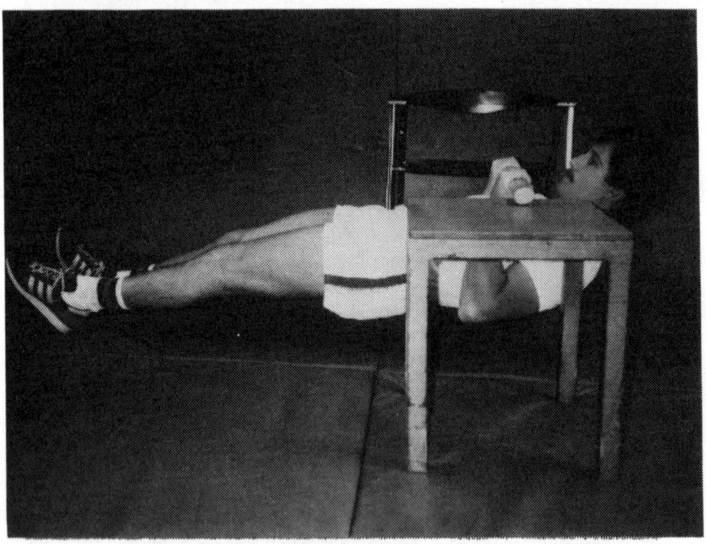

Inclined Press-Ups – Shoulder girdle, Extensors of Elbow, Upper Chest, Tummy. (Isotonic).
With both feet supported on a chair or similar, body inclined downwards, supported by the hands. Bend and stretch the elbows. Exercise may be intensified by raising the feet even higher.
(Isometric). Stand in a door frame, raise the arms and press upwards against the lintel, holding pressure for approximately six seconds. Use something to stand on if necessary. (Does not activate tummy muscles).

FIGURE 22

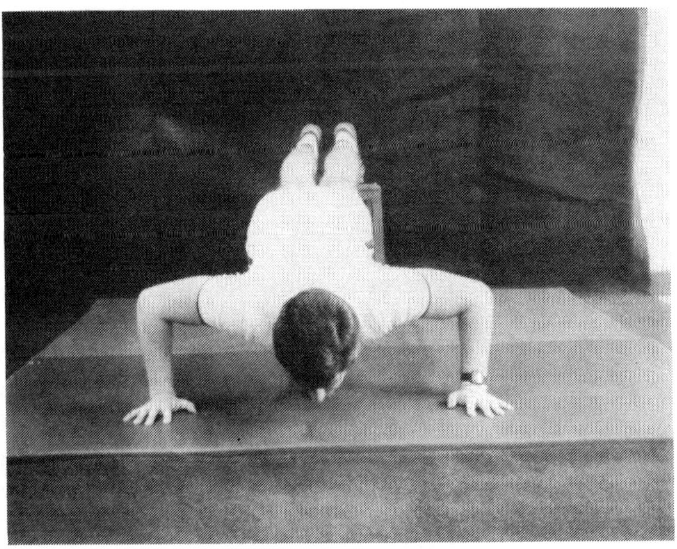

(Opposite) **Bicep Curls** – Flexors of Elbow.
(Isotonic).
These can be carried out quite simply by holding any heavy object in the hand, e.g. books, suit-case, dining chair, etc. throughout the execution of the exercise, in which the elbow joint is alternately flexed and extended.
(Isometric). Sitting at a desk or heavy table, grasp the underside of the working surface with both hands, then exert an upward pull and sustain for approximately eight seconds.

6. Hyperventilation: This occurs when the CO_2 level in the blood falls as a result of over breathing (see page no. 19). By breathing into a paper bag or similar, for about fifteen to twenty minutes the CO_2 level usually returns to normal, and the symptoms subside.

   Never travel without some water purification tablets or non-absorbable antacids. Have them to travel, but also at home. More extreme forms of upset stomach may cause diarrhoea or constipation and it is essential to take precautions if these extreme conditions occur.

FIGURE 23

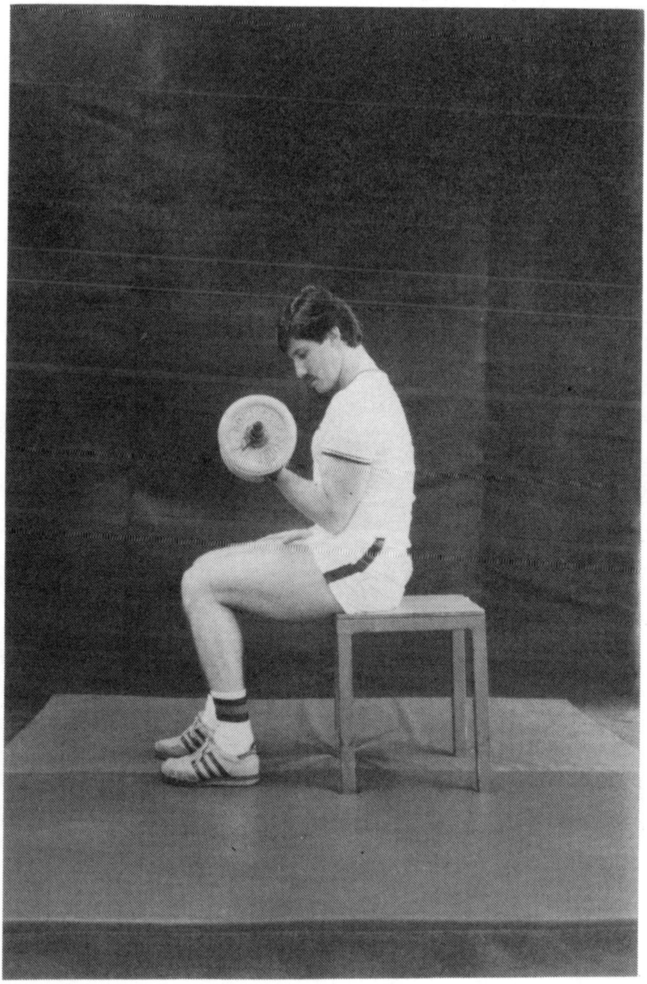

Press-Ups – Upper Chest, Extensors of Elbow, Tummy. (Isotonic).
As No. 22, but feet supported on floor. Easier form of press-up, but does not activate the shoulder girdle muscles so much.
(Isometric). With the elbows bent, and arms held at right angles to the body, press the hands firmly together. Sustain for six seconds.

FIGURE 24

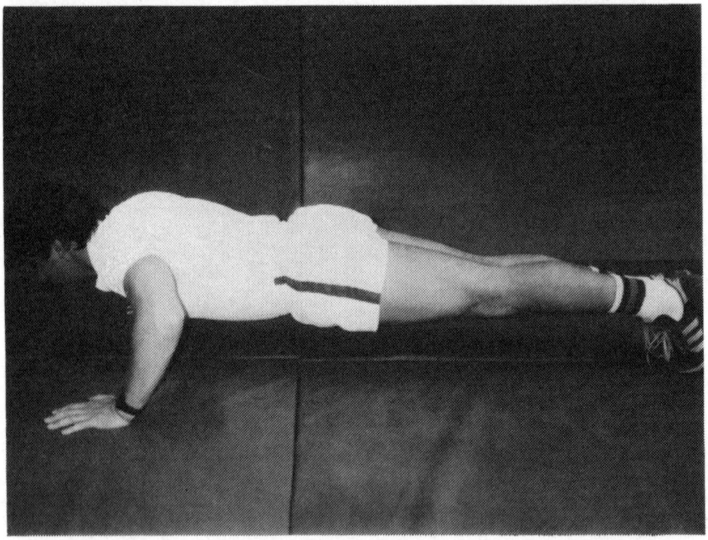

Sit-Ups – Tummy and Pelvic girdle. (Isotonic). Back lying, knees bent, feet held down, arms bent across chest or behind neck (stronger). Raise head and shoulders to bring elbow to touch opposite knee. (e.g. Right knee, to Left elbow). (Isometric). Starting position as above. Press small of back hard downwards into the floor, your tummy muscles will contract stongly. Hold contraction for approximately six seconds.

FIGURE 25

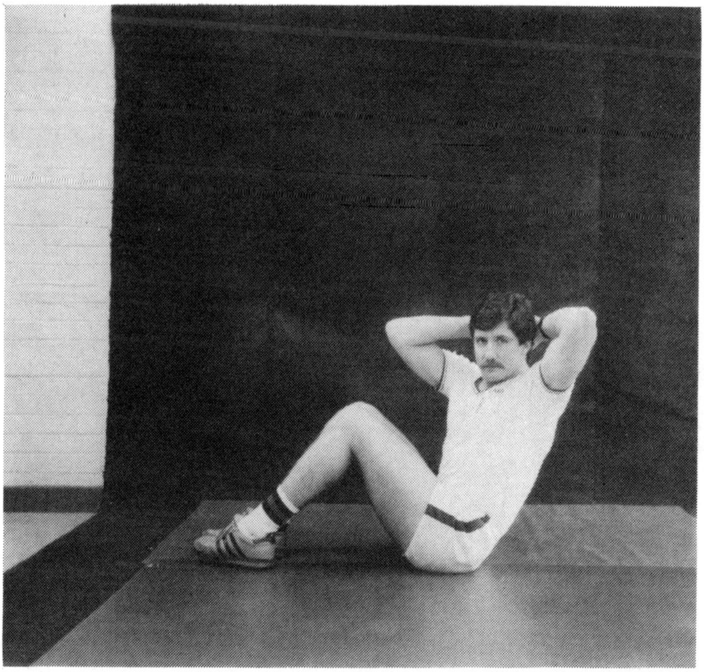

Dips – Upper Back, Extensors of Elbow, Upper Chest, Spinal Muscles. (Isotonic).
Sitting on the floor between two stools or dining chairs, place one hand on each seat. Push downwards to raise the hips keeping the heels down. The intensity of the exercise can be increased by supporting the heels at a higher level.
(Isometric). Seated in a suitable chair, i.e. one with arm supports. Place the hands on the arm rests and push downwards. Do not allow the seat to rise.

FIGURE 26

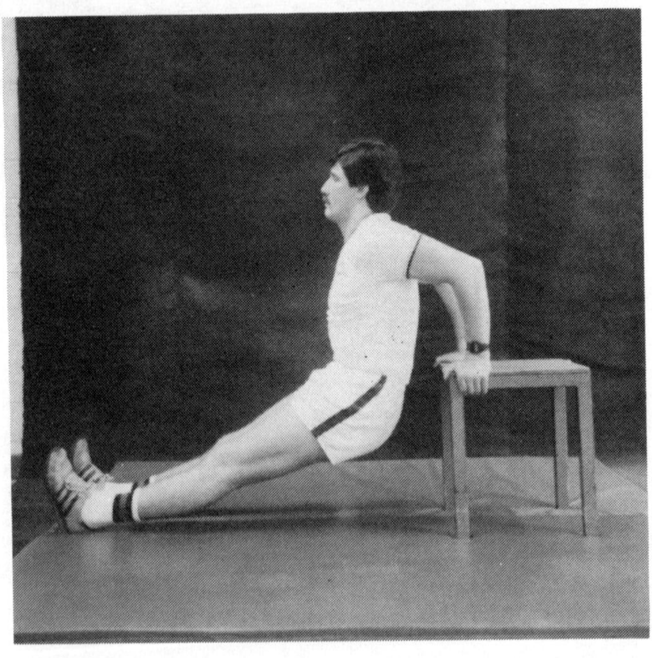

Hip and Spinal Stretch – Hamstrings, Spine, Buttocks. (Isotonic).
Back lying, knees bent, feet resting on floor, arms at sides. Raise hips as high as possible, then lower. Keep the shoulders and feet in contact with the floor during the exercise.
(Isometric). Lie on the back, press hard down on the floor with heels and shoulders, squeezing buttocks together. Do not allow body to break contact with the floor. Hold for approximately six seconds.

FIGURE 27

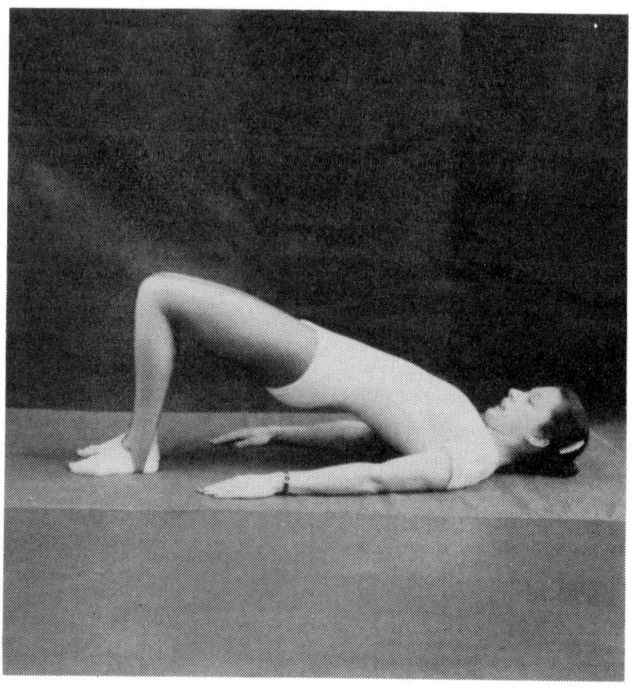

(Opposite) **Wrist Rolling** – Forearm, Grip, Wrists.
(Isotonic).
A short length of wood, or a metal rod around which is secured a length of cord attached to a weighty object, e.g. a book or document case, provides the means to perform wrist rolling. This is done by twisting the stick horizontally, using both hands, thus raising the weight. The repetitions should alternate between wrist flexion and wrist extension.
(Isometric). This, to some extent, can be achieved by squeezing a squash ball or similar held in the grip.

FIGURE 28

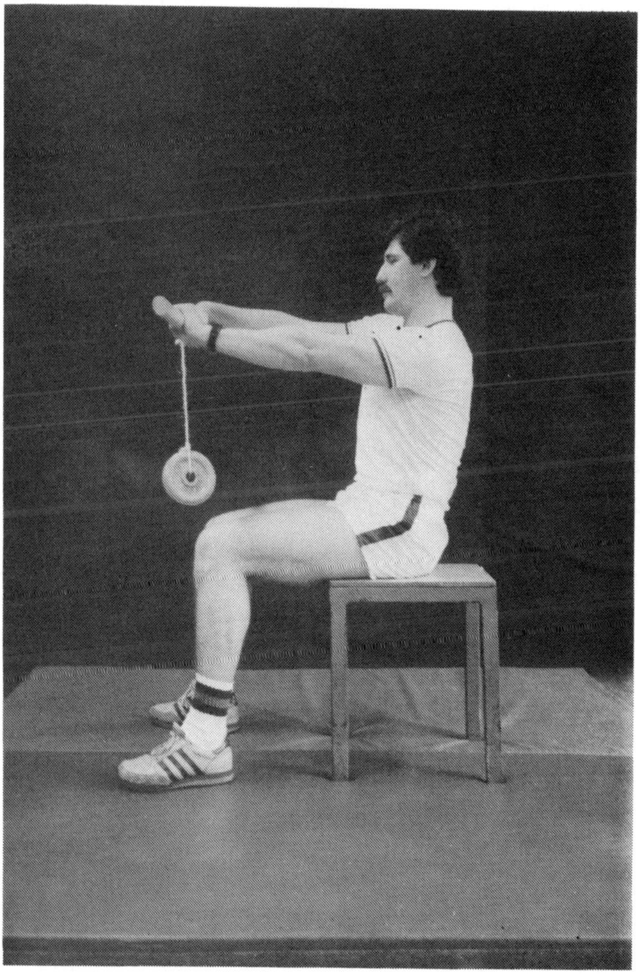

(Opposite) **Single Leg Squats** – Pelvic girdle, thigh, buttock. (Isotonic).
Sit on stool or chair, arms folded, raise one leg clear of the floor. Attempt to stand up on supporting leg five or six times before changing legs.
(Isometric). Sitting, one leg raised to the horizontal, knee flexed to approximately 140°, foot placed against stout wall. Push hard with the foot, making sure that your stool does not shift backwards.

The number of repetitions of each exercise depends on the fitness level of the participant. In the case of one who may be completely out of condition, start with four and increase by two each succeeding week.

FIGURE 29

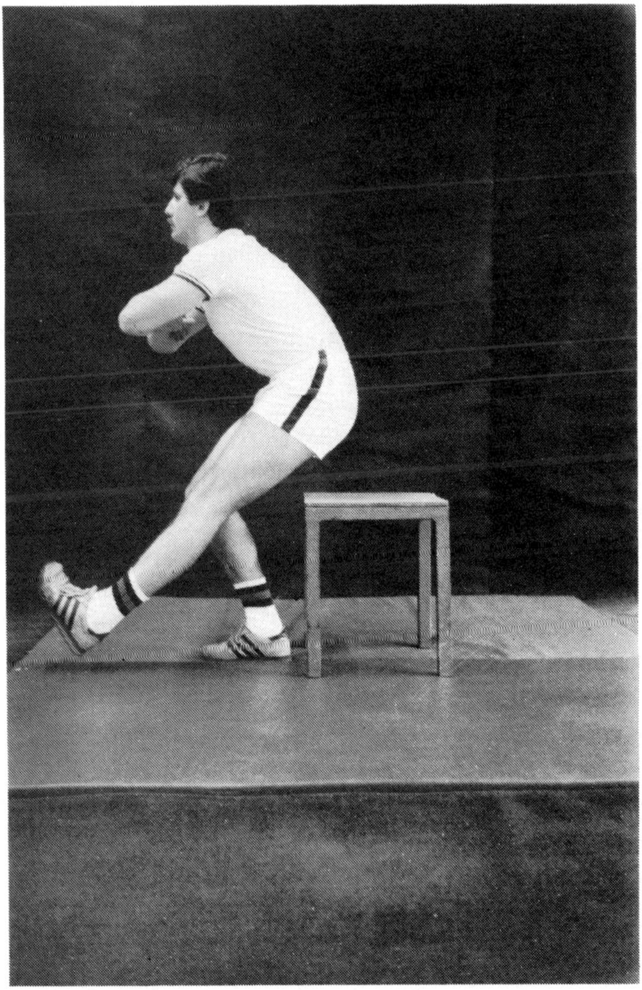

Dangerous Exercises

The chassis of your car, and its shock absorbers and suspension, are so designed that they will safely support the vital component parts unless subjected to frequent overload. This is no less true of the body's skeleton with its ligaments and cartilages. Most exercises are potentially dangerous if performed incorrectly. But some movements are, in themselves, direct contributors to abnormal stresses, and, if continued, will eventually lead to malfunction. It is unfortunate that many of these so-called 'exercises' are favourites among enthusiasts of 'physical jerks'.

Toe-touching. If performed with the knees straight, and even worse, with a rapid bouncing action, causes tremendous strain on the regions of the lower spine. This very often contributes to sciatica, and/or lower back pain. A referred pain may be felt in the buttocks or down the back of the thigh.

Sit-ups. With straight knees, is almost the same movement as above performed in the horizontal plane. It is recommended that, if performed as an exercise, the movement is rendered safe simply by bending the knees to about 90° and that the spinal column is not brought to maximum flexion.

Back lying, straight leg lifting. When lifting both legs simultaneously from a back lying position, once again a strong pull is exerted on the structures of the lower spine at the start of the movement. This causes a momentary increase in the forward curvature of the spine, resulting in possible injury. Performed with knees bent to approximately 90° throughout the movement, it becomes a safe abdominal exercise.

Deep knee squats. When the buttocks are brought down to touch the heels, the ligaments of the knee joints are stretched to their maximum. The weight of the body tends to press the articular surfaces of the joints together causing an abrasive action to occur. The degree of knee flexion in this exercise should be limited to 100°.

Prone lying, back arching. Excellent as an exercise if performed with arms assisting the raising of the shoulders. Otherwise the small posture-maintaining muscles of the spine are subjected to overload causing backache.

All movements, performed in a jerky forceful manner. This inevitably causes overstretch of the tissues surrounding the joints. Paradoxically perhaps, it causes shortening of some muscles, resulting in disharmony of development. Young girls who spent a lot of time doing arm-flinging sideways, repeating the ditty, 'I must, I must increase my bust' were, in fact, encouraging the opposite.

Post-stretch (Warm-down exercises)

At the end of your general fitness programme you are aware that you have undertaken a period of heavy activity through the stages of pre-stretch, flexibility, aerobics and power activities.

It is not advisable to stop this level of activity suddenly and that is why the post-stretch exercises are recommended at the end of the programme.

The reason that it is inadvisable to stop suddenly on a high level of activity is that it may result in the collection of blood at the body extremities (head, feet, hands). Because of the depletion of blood to the rest of the body the muscles may have an excess build-up of lactic acid and also a depletion of CO_2 which causes stiffness if not properly counterbalanced.

The procedure to avoid stiffness is to carry out the following post-stretch exercises.

Exercise 1: Lying supine, arms stretched beyond your head. Arch your spine, stretching hands and feet away. Hold for 10 seconds, repeat three times.

FIGURE 30

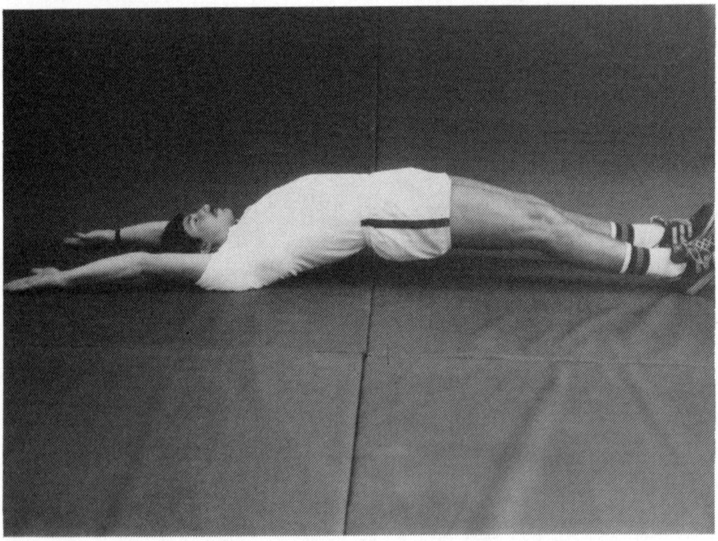

Exercise 2: Kneeling, sitting back between your feet, hands supporting. Slowly lower your shoulders backwards until a stretch is applied to the front of both thighs. Hold for 10 seconds, repeat three times.

FIGURE 31

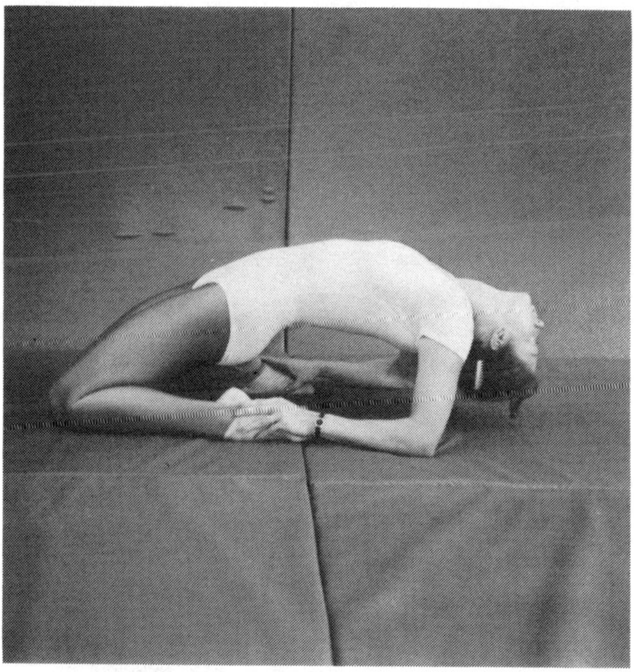

Exercise 3: Standing, one leg crossed in front of the other. Gently reach downwards pressing the knees backwards, until stretch is applied to the back of the leg. Hold for 10 seconds, repeat with each leg 3 times.

FIGURE 32

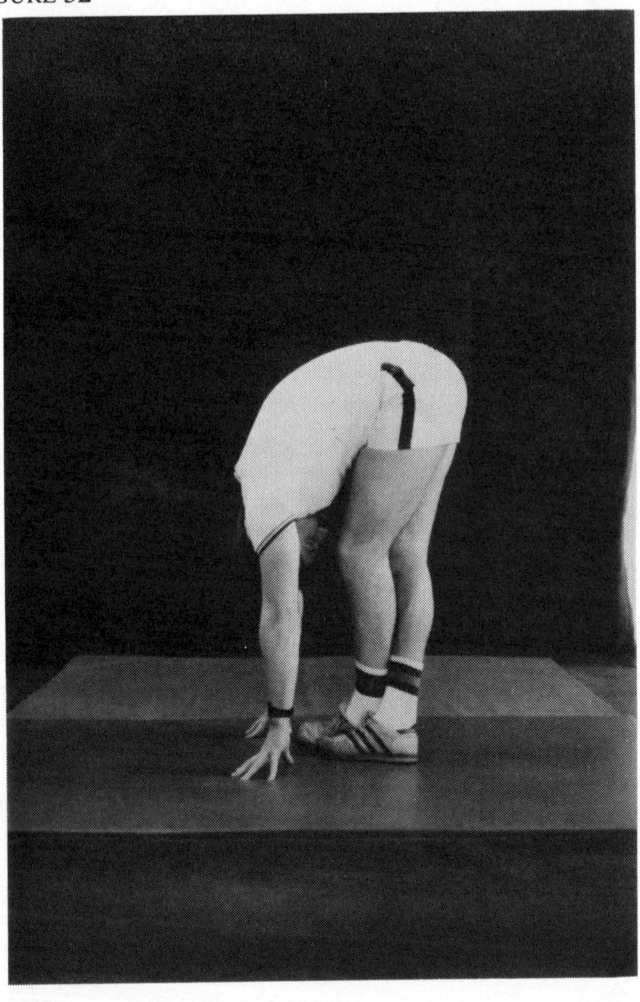

Working Out in the Home, Office or Hotel

'The whole world is a gymnasium.' Providing you have access to showers or other means of washing, it is quite easy to maintain a fitness programme by using the principles of circuit training.

Circuit training is a simple method of combining muscular endurance with aerobic benefit either of which may be given priority by the appropriate choice of exercises. The programme content may be designed to relate to individual needs. Because it is flexible, it tends to be less monotonous than many other systems, and yet it can provide an all-round development programme. The amount of space required depends upon the selection of exercises and the importance, or not, of specialised apparatus.

When designing the circuit of activity for a general fitness work-out, one should consider the five basic elements of fitness, these all begin with the letter 'S' so should be simple to remember. They are, in no particular order of importance, Stamina, Strength, Suppleness, Speed and Skill. The ingredients, in terms of exercises to give variation and to cover the five elements, are all in this book.

Select a certain number of exercises to meet your needs, then pre-determine the number of repetitions that is in line with your fitness level, for each exercise. Commence with pre-stretch and end with post-stretch exercises. In your work-out, you achieve aerobic benefit by passing rapidly from one exercise to the next, and so on, until the number of desirable circuits is performed. To allow lactic acid build-up in muscle groups to disperse between each exercise, jog on the spot for about 15 seconds, at a rate consistent with the maintenance of your training pulse-rate. Remember to do this between each of the selected exercises.

Here is an example of a circuit-training programme for an average fit man or woman of between 25 and 45. The exercises chosen may all be modified for the less fit or for older people. The only apparatus required is a stool or stout chair. There are eight exercises and each one should be repeated 10 times on each of three circuits (remembering the 15 second jog between each set of 10 repetitions) and the work-out should take about 15 minutes. Obviously, for a harder work-out it is simply a matter of increasing the repetitions or the total number of circuits, and vice-versa for an easier work-out. Always start with your pre-stretch exercises. The exercises are explained and illustrated in the following pages.

At the completion of your circuit work-out check your pulse, if it is lower than your training rate, perform additional circuits. If it is higher, modify your next work-out.

With a little imagination one can change the programme content by referring to other exercises in this book which may be more suitable to one's individual needs. Remember of course to perform your pre-stretch exercises before your circuit, and complete your work-out with warm-down if time permits.

Sit-ups: These should always be performed with the knees bent to about 90° and with feet supported. Each elbow should be brought across to touch the opposite knee.

FIGURE 33

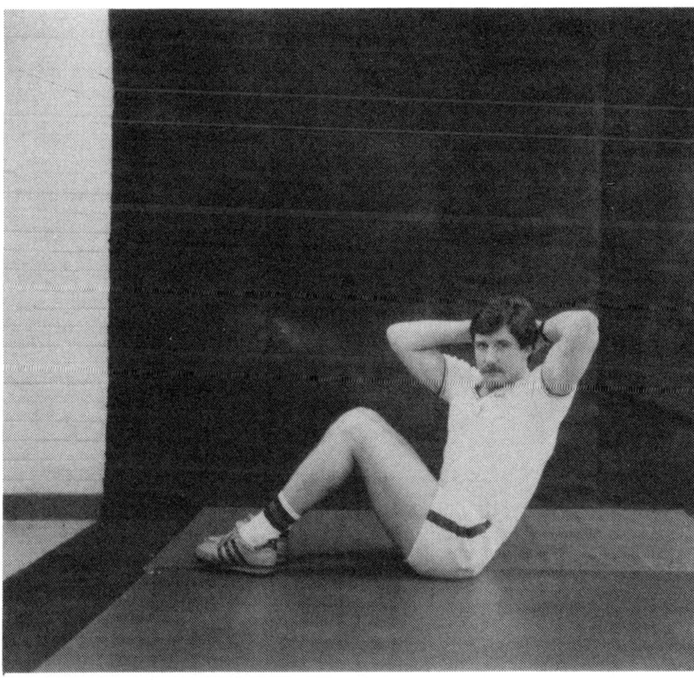

Modification shown.

FIGURE 34

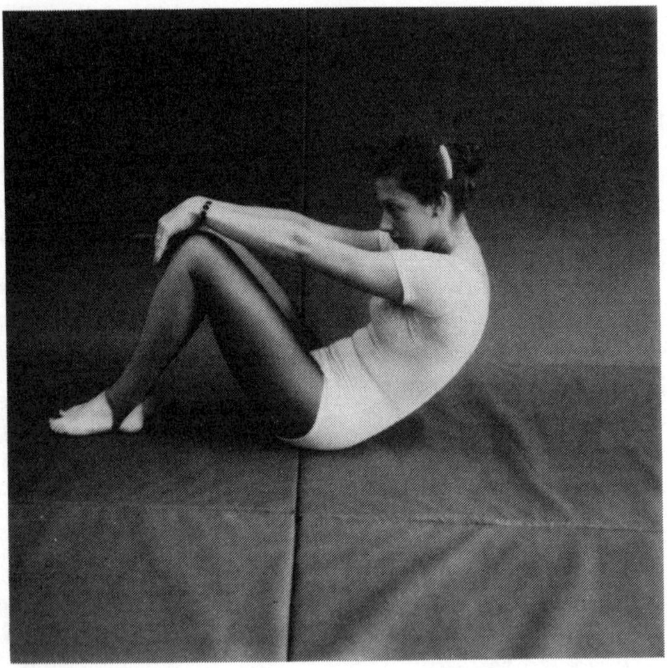

Squat thrusts: From a front support position, legs straight, bring both knees up between the arms together, then shoot back to starting position. Modify by bending the knees alternately to squat position.

FIGURE 35

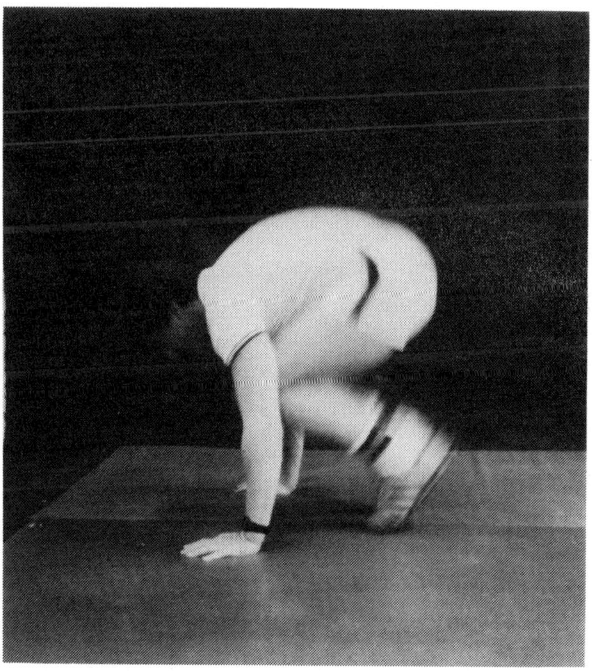

(Opposite) **Rotations:** Stand with back to stool or chair, legs astride, keeping the feet as fixed as possible, twist around to pick up chair with both hands, crossing in front replace chair and twist the other way. Repeat exercise 5 times each direction. Modify by using an object, such as a pillow or book on top of the chair, lift the object and twist to replace on the chair.

FIGURE 36

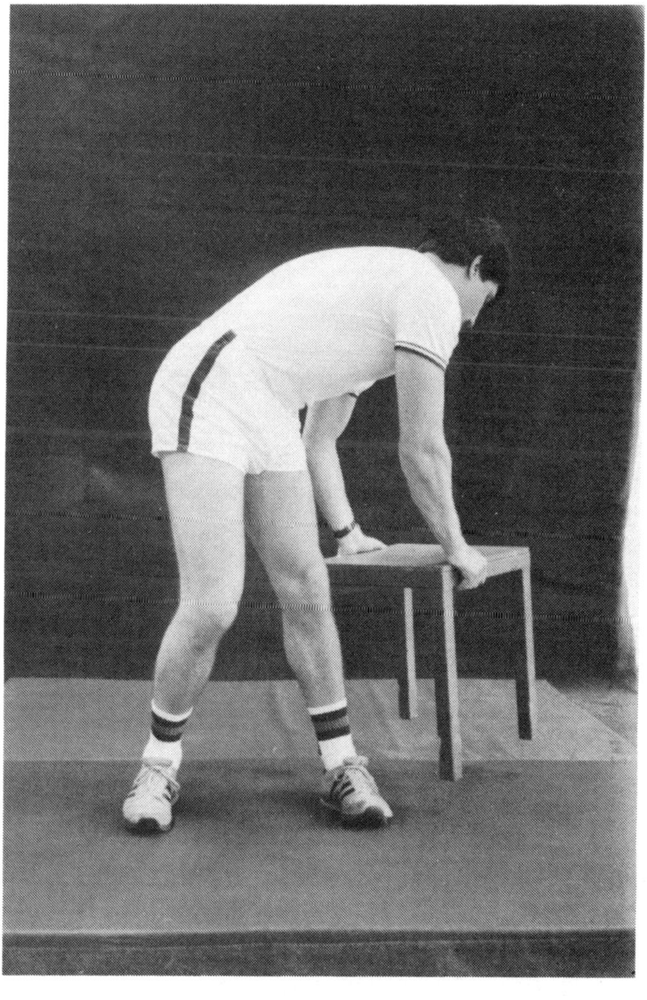

Scissors: Lying on back arms stretched beyond the head. Raise one leg to about 60° at the same time reach forward with both hands, raising the head and shoulders, touch foot, then return to starting position to repeat other side. Keep knees straight throughout unless a modification is required when knees may be bent.

FIGURE 37

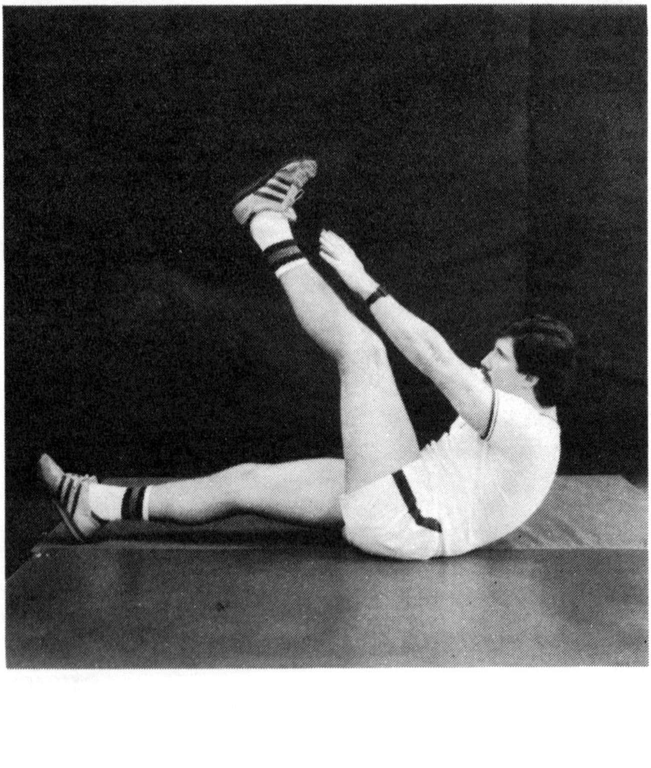

Step-ups: These are performed as explained for fitness test, page 24. Modify by using hand support such as cupboard top.

FIGURE 38

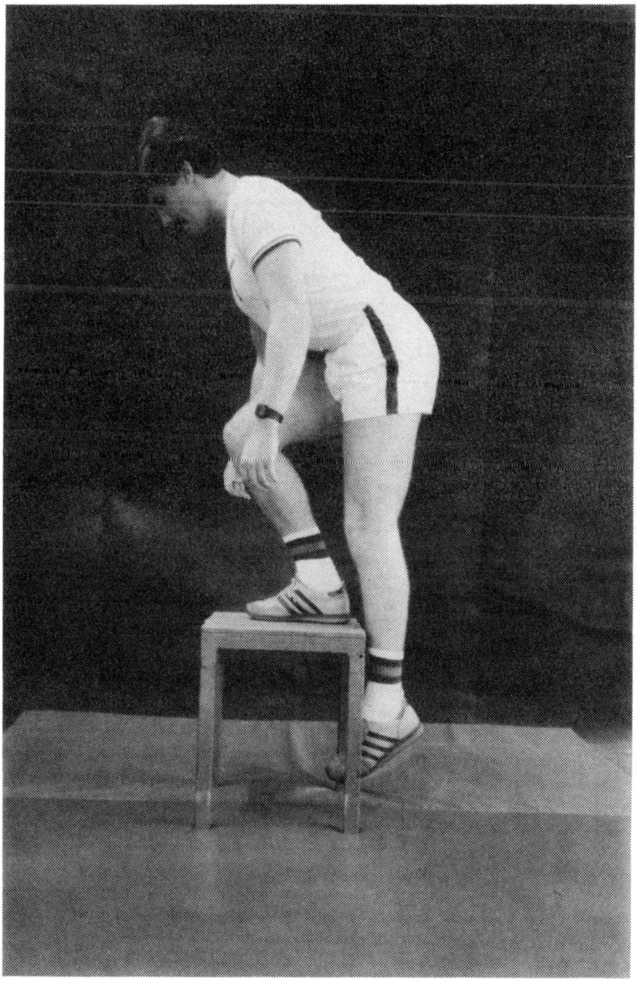

Press-ups: From a front support position, legs and hips straight, bend both arms together until the chest is about 4 inches from the floor, then return to starting position.

FIGURE 39

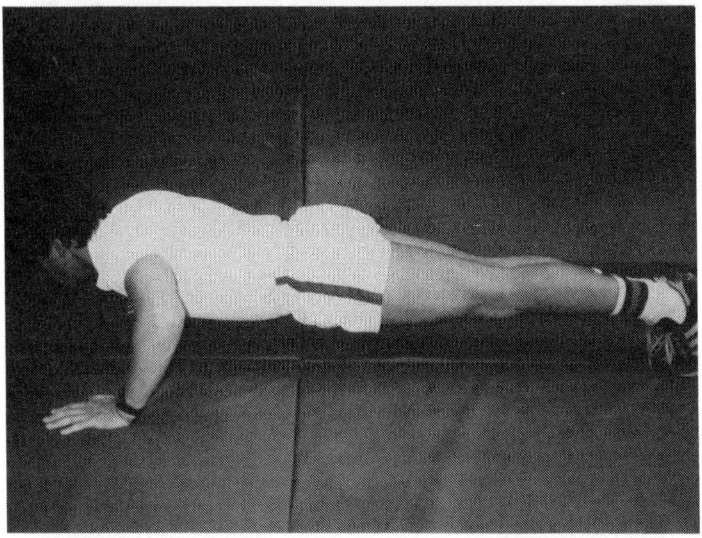

Modify by using half press-up or 'seal'.

FIGURE 40

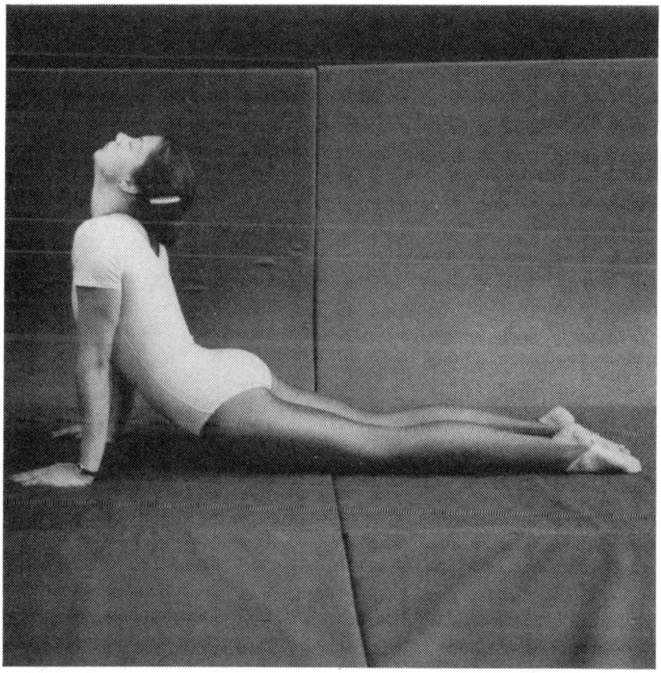

Tuck-jumps: Standing, spring up bending both knees as high onto the chest as possible. Modify by using *alternate* high knee raise.

FIGURE 41

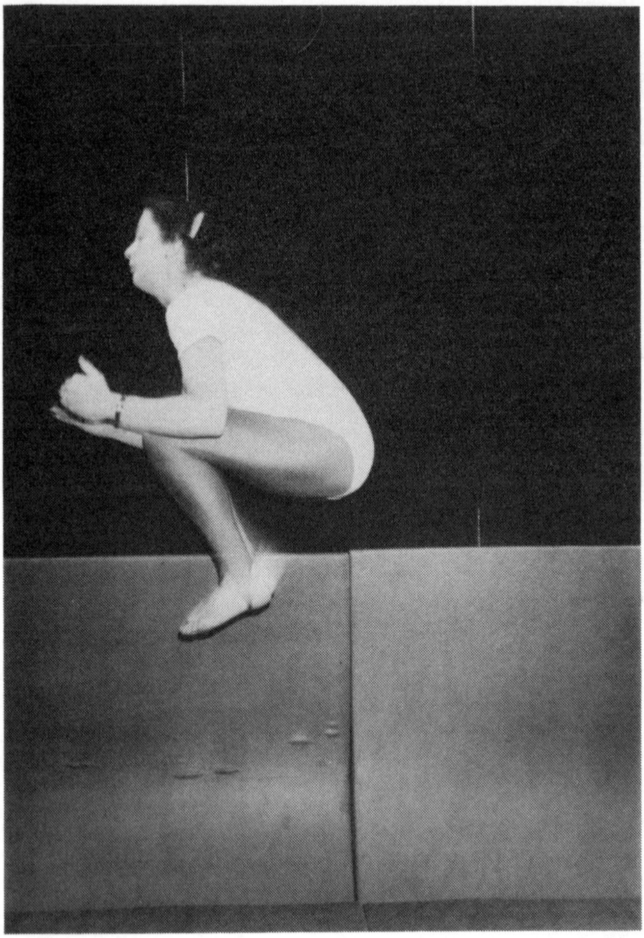

Dips: With your back to the chair, hold on to the chair seat with both hands. Lower your hips as far as the elbow bend will allow, then return to raise the hips as high as possible. Modify by performing the exercise at floor level, dispensing with chair.

FIGURE 42

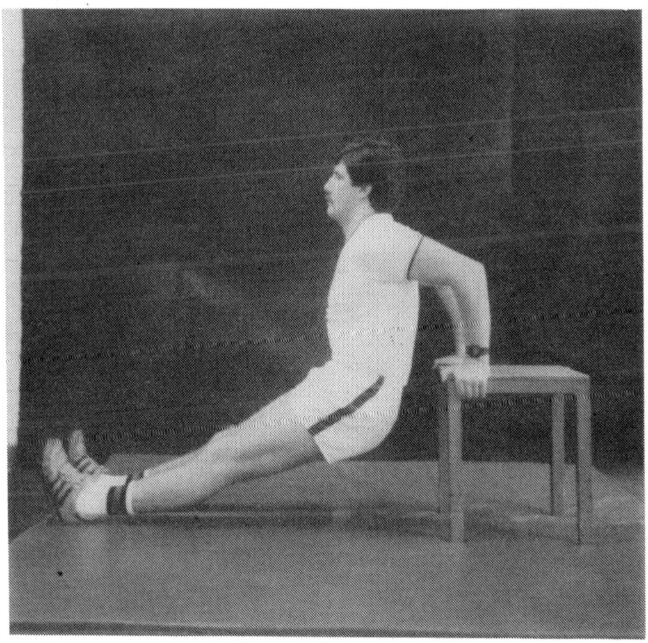

Travelling

The general fitness exercises to be carried out in the home, office or hotel have already been outlined. It is possible to carry out a daily fitness routine wherever one happens to be. However, the pressures and difficulties encountered when travelling really do test the ingenuity and dedication of the executive fitness aficionado.

Family, friends and colleagues often ask about the exotic places executives visit. The well travelled executive can rarely say much about the more commercial and cultural aspects of the cities throughout the world. Ask him about the airline clubs, his favourite airline, duty free shops, the most efficient mode of getting to and from airports, where to get a quick snack or drink and he will confound you with his intricate knowledge. It is all directed at speed, turnaround time and perhaps getting back to the family or office as soon as possible. Outside of these environs executives rarely spend time exploring the locality visited unless there is an extended meeting or conference where there is adequate time free for doing your own thing. The effect of the obsession with getting there quickly, doing the job in a hurry and returning post haste sets up certain pressures and temptations.

Pressures of travel: The pressures start at the planning stage. Tickets, currency, passport (with relevant visa) correct shots depending on which country is being visited, car booked at this and the other end, the itinerary, up-to-date briefing and presentations, current credit cards and relevant driving licence and insurance cover. These aspects of travel are generally efficiently carried out by the secretary. However, the many variables involved frequently mean some kind of a 'screw-up'. The result is that, before the executive leaves the office either to drive or get driven to the airport, he has begun to set up stress and anxiety levels on some aspect of the travel schedule. The journey to the airport can be quite hair-raising on occasions. Nose-to-tail traffic when you give a driver thirty minutes for a forty-five minute journey. If you drive yourself you arrive at your favourite parking lot to find the FULL sign prominently displayed. When being driven you can work contentedly, but can you when the driver is taking a route not familiar, which is bound to be longer and doubts begin to arise as to whether or not you'll make the check-in time?

The widely travelled executive is the master of travelling light – he knows all the tricks of 'one piece of hand luggage' which can range from a document folder to the three-in-one case; somehow or another they all fit under the seat.

More hassle at the airport; baggage handlers on strike, flights delayed because of weather, technical defects, changes due to lack of utilisation of aircraft, catering is delayed, or insufficient, the passengers on the previous flight drank all the booze.

The car or bus journey on arrival can be fraught with problems – only travellers cheques, no local currency? Arrive at the hotel to find it fully booked – no, there was no confirmation of your stay. Yes, there is a swimming pool but it's empty this time of year or it's undergoing maintenance. The executive is used to these minor problems and has an enormous capacity to fob them off and put them down to experience. However, there is a breaking point for everyone and we all have our pet stories. Mine is being fog bound in Paris and taking two and a half days to get back to London, by train and boat – a marathon sleepless feat with no time to spend on training at any stage of the journey.

It is highly desirable when you have arrived at your destination to devote adequate time for relaxation and circuit training. Build this into your schedule beforehand and suprisingly you will get it accomplished.

Temptations of travel: Prevention is by far the best course of action for the fitness fanatic. Moderation is advocated for our readers.

What are the different things available when travelling?

Arrival at the airport means that you have half an hour to an hour before the flight, perhaps more if it is delayed. Ensconced in the airline club you are exposed to free drinks, sandwiches and biscuits to soothe your nerves – after a rough time getting this far. You have time to visit the duty free shop for booze, cigars, cigarettes and those wonderful chocolates for family, friends, whoever happens to be lucky enough to be on the receiving end, this trip. In-flight meals and drinks: the better the class of travel the greater the obesity load becomes. How about on arrival? You will often be met by colleagues and whisked off to a lengthy dinner meeting; of course you have to sample the local fare. This includes delicacies across the whole range of food and drink depending on the season.

You have been exposed to three lots of drinks, two snacks and a full blown meal and you haven't unpacked yet. There is no need to imbibe all three, although it is difficult to forego everything particularly if you are accompanied or being entertained. There is nothing to stop you drinking non-alcoholic drinks, however, and this is to be encouraged as it helps to prevent dehydration during the flight.

Pressures continue during the stay with 'fat-loading'. The stress and accompanied hassle start up again on the return journey.

Precautions when travelling: Never travel without giving some thought to the following:

1. The effect of cold drinks
2. Ice in your drinks

3. Local water
4. Sunburn
5. Upset stomach
6. Constipation and diarrhoea
7. Change in food

It is quite simple to have a relatively small medical kit which will quickly allay most of the common problems associated with travelling. As you will appreciate you know your metabolism better than anyone else. A little thought on moderation and providing the right cures will see you through.

Aches and pains when travelling: The ride in the car, lying back in the lounge, cramped up in the plane will sometimes lead to aches and pains. What about the overnight flight? It is recommended that you walk around the aircraft, if possible, to keep the circulation going – or you can just do some isometric exercises to keep the blood flow going. (Please refer to page 68 onwards.)

Jet lag when travelling: One of the more frequent problems executives face is jet lag. This seems to vary in its impact from one person to another. It is inadvisable to drive after a six to eight hour flight, although many people do.

Always take your running shoes when travelling and keep up your fitness programme. There is nothing more spectacular than jogging in far away places such as the beaches of Hawaii, the Caribbean, the forest trails of the Nordic countries and Germany, the splendour of Athens and far flung places too numerous to mention. It is quite amazing that most places in the Americas, Europe, Middle and Far East and Australasia have magnificent facilities to support keeping fit. Apart from the stresses, temptations and local problems there is no excuse to put off your training when travelling.

The Back Problem

Disorders of the lower back are more and more prevalent in today's society. Lack of exercise, with poor muscle tone and bad posture, combined with the stresses imposed by a modern life-style, serve to predispose individuals to acute back problems which often tend to recur and eventually become chronic.

The person with various anatomical weaknesses, congenital or acquired, in the low back region is prone to acute pain. The individual with poor abdominal musculature or faulty vertebral alignment with its associated muscle imbalance and lack of soft-tissue extensibility has all the ingredients for future injury and chronic low back pain. An increased forward curvature of the lower spine is very often either the result of, or associated with, tight musculature in the same area, with a concomitant weakness of the abdominal muscles, which often causes a forward pelvic tilt. This condition is characterised by a sagging of the waist line with a gravitational pull on the abdomen. It should not be surprising that this consistent strain eventually causes pain and instability in the lower back. Perhaps this is why, during the latter weeks of pregnancy, women experience pain in the loins.

It would appear that, to overcome the constant gravitational downward and forward pull on unsupported tissue, the individual needs to arch his spine, and this results in muscle tension. The pain is usually insidious in onset and is often referred to as postural backache.

To try and correct these irregularities, one must attack the weakened muscle groups and remobilise the affected segments of the spine. It is to a large extent true that the exercises that follow contribute to improved general posture, thus serving more than one useful purpose. It is important to remember that these exercises are not designed to aggravate the conditions! Therefore, apart from the usual slight muscle soreness experienced after exercising new muscle groups, any movements that increase back pain should be stopped immediately.

There have been many words written on the subject of posture, most of them on methods to correct bad postural habits of a lifetime. These methods are probably successful if carried out conscientiously for many months and provided that permanent skeletal changes have not taken place. However, many of the business people with low back pain and cervical symptoms are victims, not of permanent bad posture but of periods throughout the working day when they adopt postures that (because of muscle imbalance and uneven pressures) give rise to pain. It is important to understand that the simple answer to the problem may just be a change of chair, or the placing of a telephone at a different height.
The simple rules are:

STAND TALL, WALK TALL, SIT TALL.

Adjust working surfaces to prevent stooping.
Avoid long periods in static positions, e.g. long journeys without a stretch.
Sleep and sit on firm supporting surfaces.
Buy a new set of clothes, it's surprising how they enhance bearing!

General mobilising exercises

In the ideal situation mobilising exercises take the form of recreational activity geared to the level of ability. Such games as Table-Tennis, Padder-Tennis, Quoits, as well as some pair activities using sticks and balls, are excellent remobilisation exercises. However, a few specific mobilisation exercises may help to supplement your programme and are useful means of measuring progress.

Rotation

Position: Back lying legs apart, arms out at 90°. Palms uppermost.

Execution: Reach across with one hand to touch opposite hand, repeat each side.

Note: heels should remain in contact with supporting surface, elbows should be kept straight throughout.

FIGURE 43

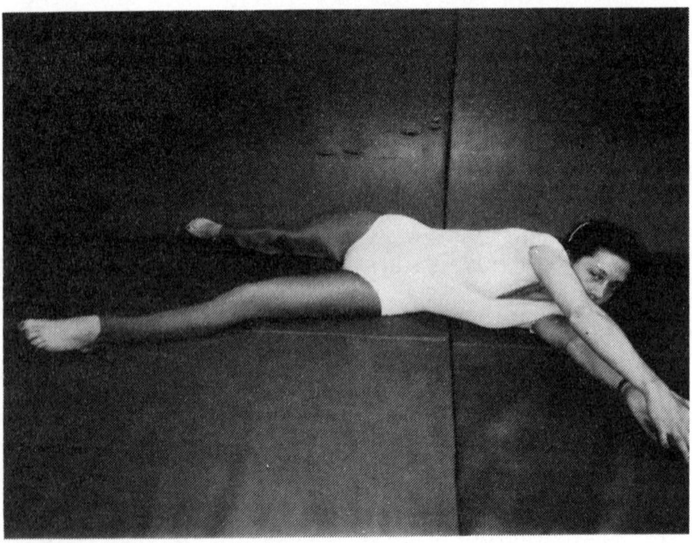

Rotation

Position: Back lying, knees bent, feet resting on supporting surface, arms out at 90° palms down.
Execution: Rock knees from side to side as far as possible.
Note: keep knees together throughout.

FIGURE 44

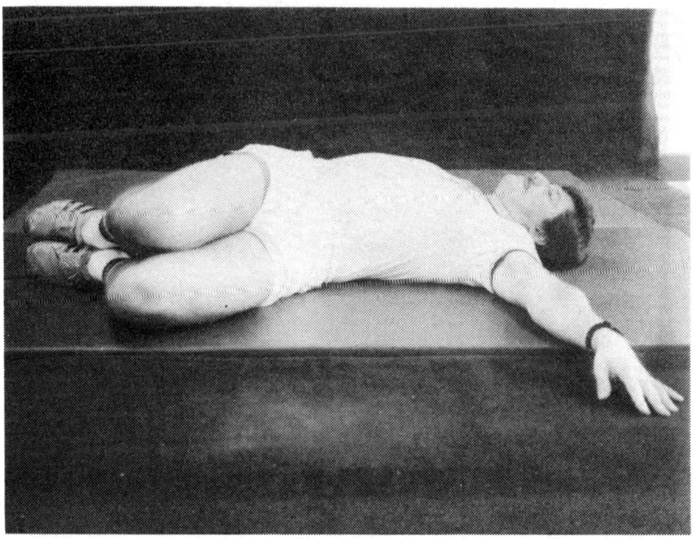

Hip Extension

Position: Back lying, knees bent, feet resting on supporting surface. Arms at side, palms down.

Execution: Raise hips as high as possible, keeping shoulders in contact with supporting surface.

FIGURE 45

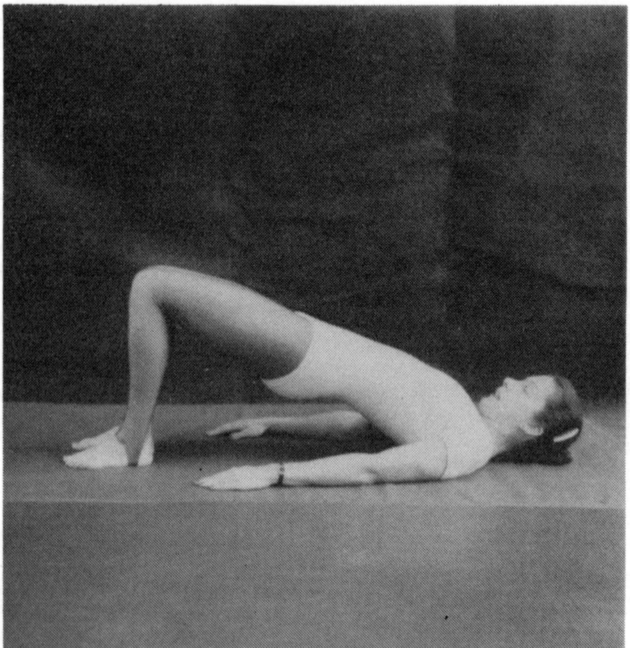

Rotation with Flexion
Position: Standing, feet astride, arms hanging loosely.
Execution: Try to touch outside of the opposite knee, reaching across the body.
Note: Try to avoid flexing at the hips.

FIGURE 46

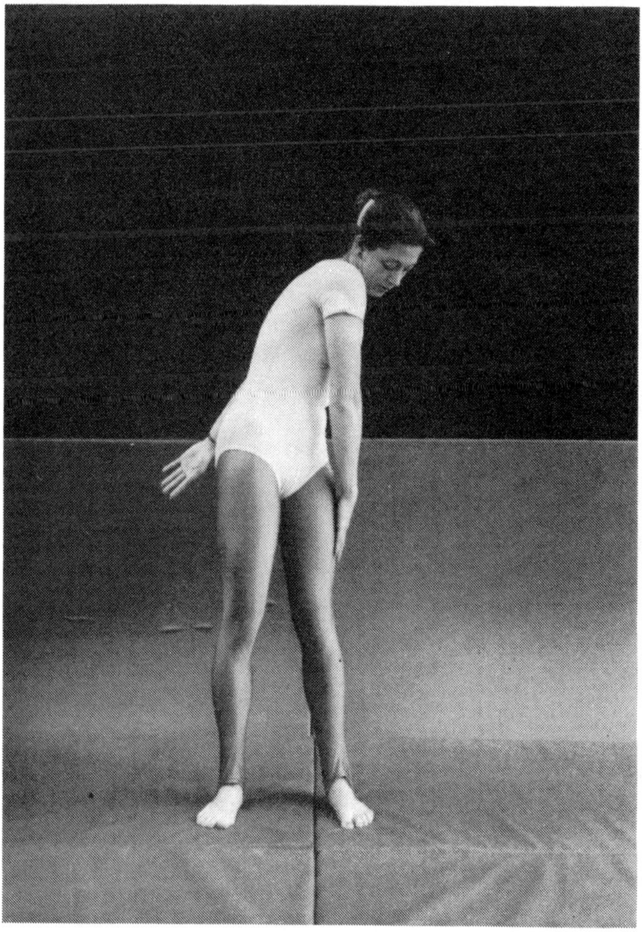

Rotation with Extension
This exercise is performed as the one above except that the reach is made *behind* the body towards the *back* of the opposite knee.

FIGURE 47

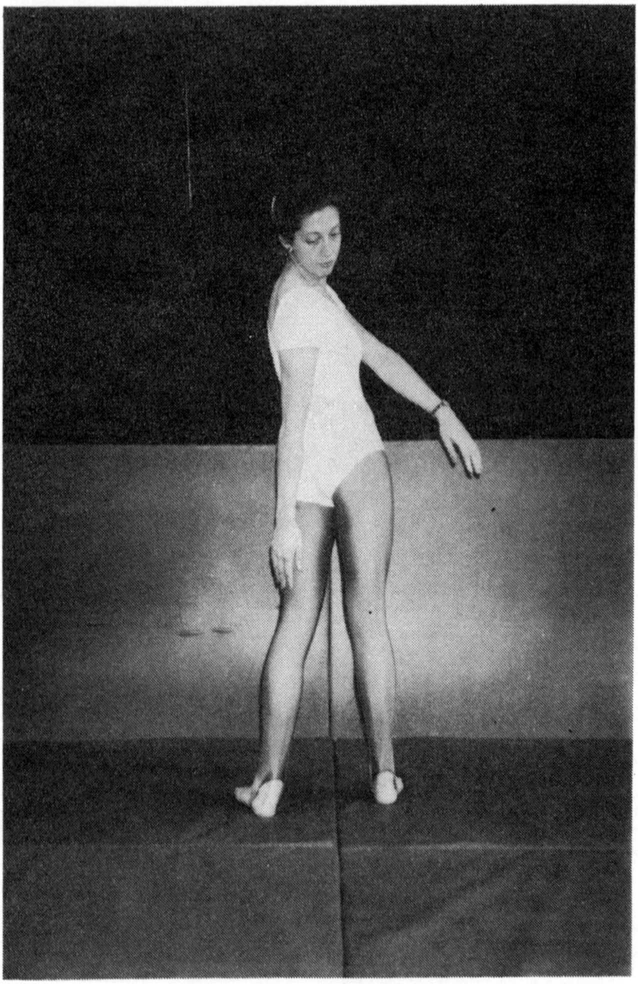

Flexion

These exercises are the same as those outlined in the section for Low Back stretch, which follow.

Low Back Stretching

Anyone with an exaggerated foward spinal curve often finds it difficult to round the back fully. A safe method to increase forward flexion can be carried out from the back lying position.

(Opposite) Variations of safe forward flexion, and an exercise which often gives rapid increase to muscle extensibility is performed by the person supporting the weight of the upper part of his body on his hands, which are placed on a raised platform or seat top, this position is taken up from a full knee bend, start with the spine held straight. The knees are now slowly straightened, causing the spine to flex forward, but with support from the arms. Forward flexion can be slowly increased by lowering the platform height until flexion of the hips is incorporated into the movement, and so long as the range of movement is pain-free.

FIGURE 48

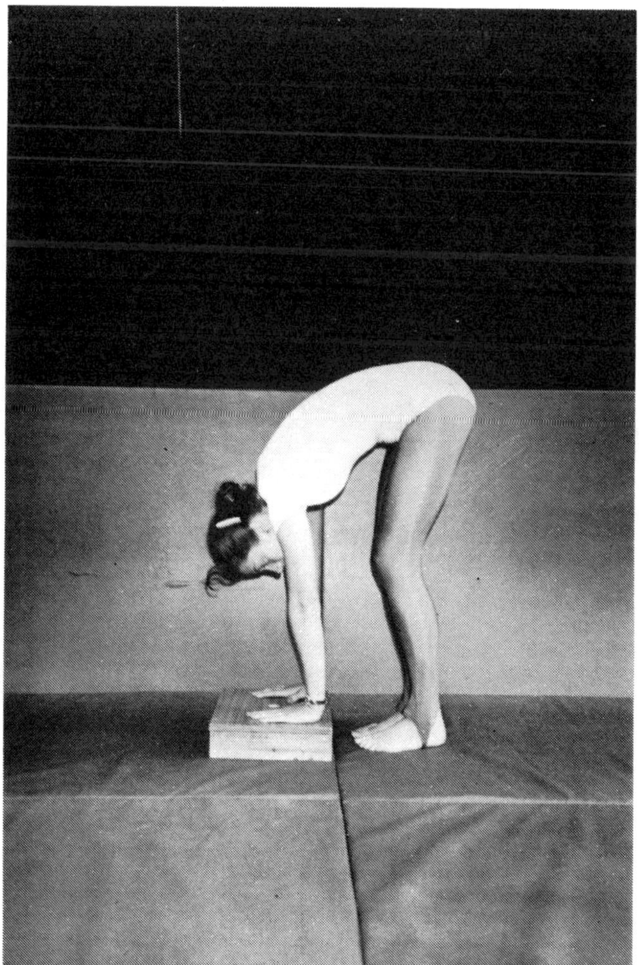

The knees are first pulled alternately to the chest and then, if no undue discomfort is experienced, both knees are brought to the chest.

FIGURE 49

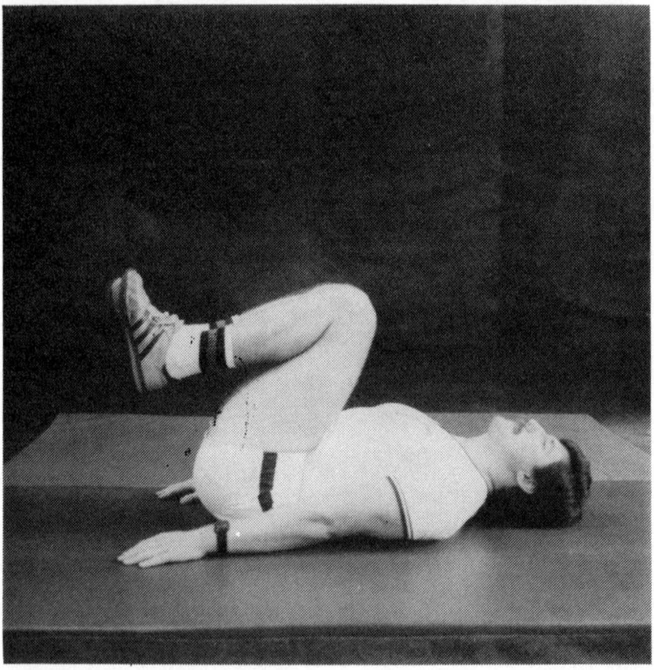

Abdominal Strengthening

All abdominal exercises should be done with the minimum strain being placed on the lumbar spine. Effective abdominal exercises can be carried out in safety by taking up the 'crook lying' position, such as one does when performing the abdominal curl. Take the crook lying position with arms extended forward. Keeping the hips and knees flexed throughout, slowly curl up the trunk.

FIGURE 50

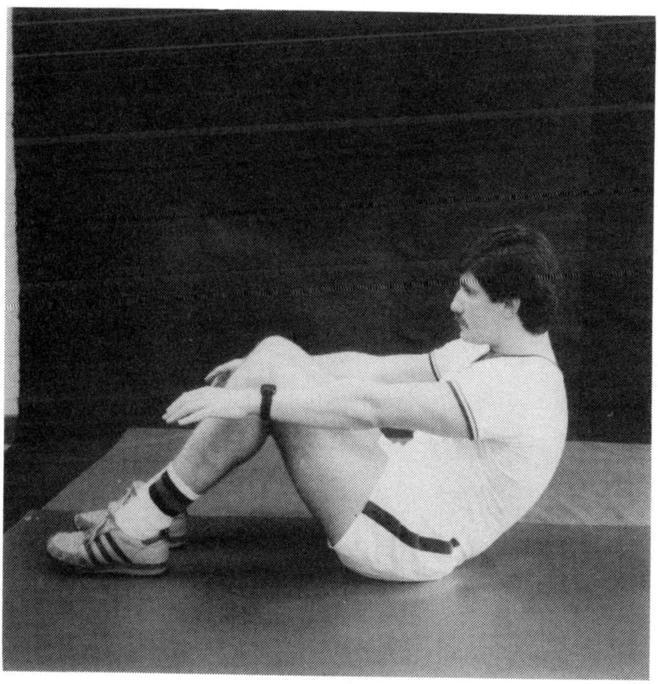

Pelvic Tilting

These are designed to strengthen the lower abdominal and pelvic floor muscles, and to stretch the lumbo-sacral muscles. Take the crook lying position. The forward spinal curvature curve is then flattened against the supporting surface by contracting the stomach muscles, this is then followed by a forward tilt of the pelvis, arching the spine from sacrum to thorax, without allowing the buttocks to lift. A contraction of the 'seat' muscles is performed during the latter part of the exercise.

FIGURE 51

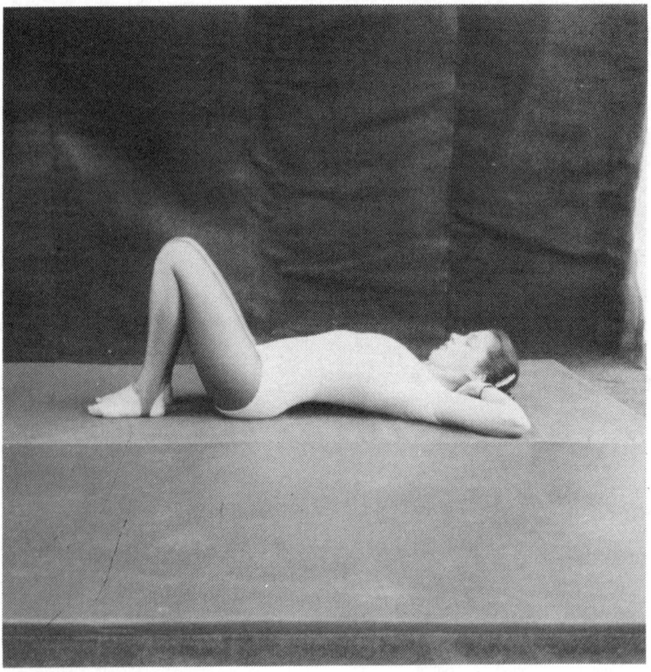

Exercises for Relaxation

Many of the obscure aches and pains of the office-bound may be due to muscular tension resulting in a build-up of metabolites in the muscle tissue. The inability of some to fully relax those muscles groups that are not actually needed during certain periods of the day is largely due to a lack of muscle identification and habitual bad posture.

Identifying abnormal tension areas can be helped by a series of exercises that cause contraction followed by relaxation of specific muscle groups. Eventually, by practice, one is able to detect those areas that require a negative muscular state, and is able to respond automatically.

In the early stages of learning relaxation it is best to practice in the supine position with comfortable support of contact areas. Later one is able to relax muscles at will in any position, and even when lying on a hard surface.

The procedure is as follows:

Use an area where there are no harsh lights or noise, make sure that you are *lying comfortably*. First of all, concentrate on your breathing, which should be gentle.

Exercise 1

Point the toes, stretching the feet, check that all other muscles are relatively relaxed. Hold for about five seconds then 'let go'. The 'letting go' is the important element in all these exercises, make sure you really 'let go'.

Exercise 2

Curl the toes, bringing the feet backwards.

Hold – 'let go'.

Exercise 3

Press the heels downwards toward the floor.

Hold – 'let go'.

Exercise 4
Tighten the thigh muscles.
Hold – 'let go'.

Exercise 5
Squeeze the cheeks of the bottom together.
Hold – 'let go'.

Exercise 6
Arch the spine.
Hold – 'let go'.

Exercise 7
Turn the legs inwards.
Hold – 'let go'.

Exercise 8
Turn the legs outwards.
Hold – 'let go'.

Exercise 9
Press small of back into floor.
Hold – 'let go'.

Exercise 10
Turn the palms of the hands upwards and press shoulders down toward the floor.
Hold – 'let go'.

Exercise 11
Check all muscles are relaxed and listen to your breathing for half a minute.
Hold – 'let go'.

Exercise 12
Push the head hard down into the pillow or floor.
Hold – 'let go'.

Exercise 13
Clench the teeth hard.
Hold – 'let go'.

Exercise 14
Check all muscles are relaxed, and try to feel a floating sensation.

Exercise 15
(See below).

It may take several practice sessions before you really begin to learn 'on the spot' muscle release; once this has been achieved it should be possible to respond automatically to muscle tension.

Exercise 15: Move slowly to adopt the 'coma position' and try to identify mentally any areas of tension. Try to relax these areas and rest.

FIGURE 52

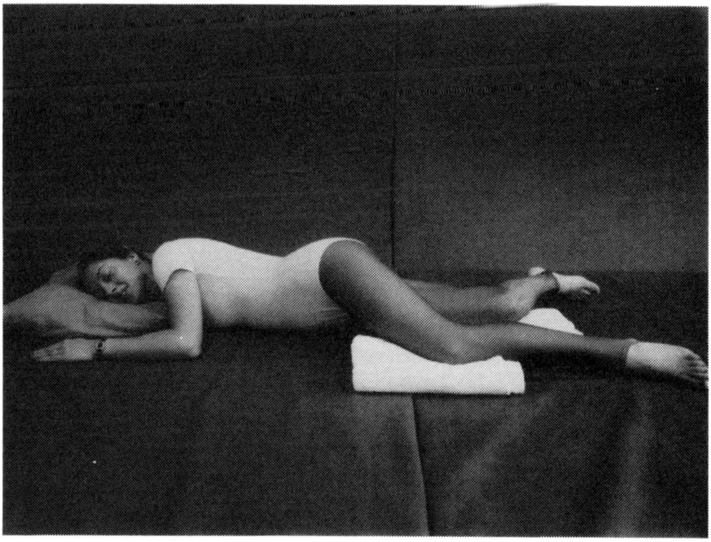

V

Par For The Course – How Do You Rate?

This chapter will outline various activities whereby you can measure, within your age category, whether or not you are below, at or above 'PAR'.

It is advisable to complete 2 to 3 weeks of the general fitness programme before assessing the level of performance.

A series of balanced exercises have been selected to measure progression related to age. They are simple and really minimise any skill needed for assessment. Once again, the emphasis is on self analysis.

The standards are not those for trained athletes, but reflect a good to high level of fitness.

The exercises incorporate a range of fitness elements including speed and agility, stamina, suppleness, strength and neuro-muscular co-ordination.

It is important that all the exercises commence with pre-stretch and end with post-stretch.

The exercises tabulated on the following page are for men, but the bottom of the table indicates how the exercises can be modified for women. A rest period of at least 2 minutes should be taken between each exercise – and at least one aerobic element should be completed, either the jogging or the cycling.

'PAR' FOR THE COURSE
HOW DO YOU RATE?

ACTIVITIES	*SUPPLENESS 30 Reps Squat Thrusts*	*STRENGTH 30 Reps Sit-Ups (feet held down)*	*STRENGTH 20 Reps Press-Ups*	*CO-ORDINATION 50 Reps Step-Ups (18" high)*	*SPEED AND AGILITY 40 Reps Hurdle-Jumps (12" high feet together)*	*AEROBICS (Endurance Minutes) 1.5 miles Jogging*	*3 miles Road Cycling (Flat)*	*3 miles Static Cycling (Light Resistance only)*	*AGE*
EXCELLENT	Less than 30 seconds	Less than 35 seconds	Less than 20 seconds	Less than 45 seconds	Less than 35 seconds	Less than 8 minutes	Less than 8 mins 45 secs	Less than 8 minutes	25-39
	30-35 secs	35-40 secs	20-28 secs	45-50 secs	35-40 secs	8-9 mins	8.45-9.30 mins	8-8.35 mins	40-55
	36-40 secs	41-45 secs	29-38 secs	51-56 secs	40-50 secs	9-10 mins	9.31-10.15 mins	8.36-9.10 mins	56-65
VERY GOOD	30-35 secs	35-40 secs	20-28 secs	45-50 secs	50-60 secs	10-11 mins	8.45-9.30 mins	8-8.35 mins	25-39
	36-40 secs	41-45 secs	29-38 secs	51-56 secs	1-1.14 mins	11-11.30 mins	9.31-10.15 mins	8.36-9.10 mins	40-55
	41-45 secs	46-50 secs	39-48 secs	57-63 secs	1.15-1.29 mins	11.30-12.30 mins	10.16-11 mins	9.11-9.45 mins	56-65
GOOD	36-40 secs	41-45 secs	29-38 secs	51-56 secs	1-1.14 mins	11-11.30 mins	9.31-10.15 mins	8.36-9.10 mins	25-39
	41-45 secs	46-50 secs	39-48 secs	57-63 secs	1.15-1.29 mins	11.30-12.30 mins	10.16-11 mins	9.11-9.45 mins	40-55
	46-50 secs	51-60 secs	49-58 secs	64-70 secs	1.30-1.45 mins	12.30-14 mins	11-12 mins	9.46-10.20 mins	56-65
MODIFICATION WOMEN PRE-TRAINING	Alternate Leg Thrusts	Arms assisted	Half Press-Ups	Stool 12" high	30 reps only Alternate Feet	Extra 1 minute Allowance	Extra 1 minute Allowance	Extra 1 minute Allowance	

TABLE 12

VI

Case Studies

In order to demonstrate that the fitness programme really works we will quote you two examples of the two hundred and fifty participants.
The first executive is a thirty-eight year old man, the second a forty-one year old woman.

Case 1. The thirty-eight year old executive fully participated in the custom and practice executive lifestyle. In addition, he had an exceptionally heavy travel schedule of 30% per annum. The demanding schedule of luncheons, dinners and meetings set up the stress, obesity, breathlessness and aches and pains we have talked about. This is the life he knew and felt relatively 'comfortable' with. But the lower back pain started to become an increasing problem, he had to rest on going up stairs and long walks demanded increased rest periods. It was obvious to his family, work associates and friends that he needed professional help. It was suggested to him that he should get advice from the professional supervisor of the fitness centre.

Awareness building:

The dialogue that ensued with the fitness supervisor was extremely positive. The executive had someone he could relate to, who could understand his problem and give him the confidence and assurance that he knew how to remedy it. The catalyst was beginning to work.

The first discussion can be summarized as follows, by both parties.

First, the subject was extremely keen to understand why he was obese and suffered from breathlessness.

Second, he wanted to learn how to put these problems right.

Third, he was prepared to be measured on achievable targets. Just like work, he said.

Fourth, he was enthused by the results and achievements demonstrated by other participants in the programme.

Finally, he agreed a timetable that was mutually acceptable.

A good start?

How much had he understood? At this stage in the awareness building programme one must put the onus on the individual. Let him assess his own fitness level, let him find the time to participate.

The questionnaire:

The questionnaire on self assessment is split into three categories. These being questions of a personal nature, health factors and job and non-job related activities.

1. Personal — AGE (38)
   WEIGHT (91 Kg)

2. Health Factors — Yes / No
   - Have you ever had a serious illness or operation?

	Yes	No
• Do you now have or have you ever had or been treated for:		
– Shortness of breath?		
– High blood pressure?		
– Pains in the chest?		
– Dizzyness/Fainting?		
– Diabetes?		
– Back pains?		

3. Job and Non-Job Related Activites

	Low	Medium	High
– How would you rate your physical activity at work?			
– How would you rate your recreational activity?			
– How would you rate your present physical level?			
– How much travelling do you do a year % (30)			
– Do you smoke? Yes/No			

From discussion around the questionnaire it became clear that he was unaware of his blood pressure, and the fact that it was a key indicator to all round health; he could not recall when it had last been recorded, or even if it was high, acceptable or low. Further probing revealed that he did not know what his ideal weight should be for his height and body-type (what *was* his body type he asked?)

At this stage of the awareness build-up, the questionnaire discussion leads naturally into, 'what tests would you give to determine my fitness level?'

It is important to give a careful outline of the tests and their duration at the outset. The careful explanation should be related to his problems, his body and general health and what improvements could be anticipated. We expect this would give added zest and motivation to rectifying the problems.

Testing Time

Prior to the actual tests being administered it is advisable to take photographs full front and side. Always useful for future reference – if you have a sense of humour!

The test falls into the following five categories, each test will record the test results of the case study.

1. Physical characteristics:
   Height (5′5″) Weight (91 kg). The total skinfold thickness (to determine body fat) was measured in four key body areas – biceps, triceps, subscapular and suprailiac. The aggregated count adjusted for body type and age was recorded at 27.2. The realisation that between 25% and 30% of your body is fat, (a better expression is clinically obese!) gears you up to start the programme right there and then.

2. Blood Pressure
   The systolic (150) and diastolic (110) was measured. The results were recorded after the man had been supine, lying in a rest position, for about 10 minutes. A total of three readings were taken. The results were explained to the executive as being very high.

Exercise and a weight control programme would reduce and eventually normalise the blood pressure.

3. Resting Pulse Rate (60)
   The executive lay down for 10 minutes to ensure total rest, relaxation and relative immobility. The pulse reading was taken by placing three fingers on the wrist below the thumb – counting the beats for one minute (15 seconds × 4). The result was interesting as this was the one reading recorded that was not abnormally high. It would be interesting to see the degree of improvement in this particular aspect. (A wry smile and a pleased look from the executive – relief?)

4. Lung function
   A standard volume cylinder was used to measure this. Forced exhalation into the cylinder registered a peak flow of 540. This was the best of three readings – it is always interesting, even after explaining the lack of resistance when one blows into a cylinder, to see the look of bewilderment if a person has not done it before. After three tries they understand that there is a degree (marginal) of technique in this particular test. Having been reassured that there is a technique in this test – the executive stores his knowledge to show dramatic improvement (?) next time around.

5. Activity capacity
   As an indication of cardio vascular endurance, running on a motorised treadmill was carried out. In this particular case the speed of the treadmill was pre-set at 4 miles per hour. The executive's pulse rate was under constant surveillance as it is considered judicious to stop activity when the pulse rate reaches 170 beats a minute.

The result was: at 4 mph a pulse rate of 168 was reached in 5 minutes. This was an extremely low endurance achievement. Here was one area where significant improvements could be expected. The second and equally important part of the test is to record the pulse rate after 5 minutes' rest, that is, the pulse recovery rate. The recording after 5 minutes was 95, which was another area to be improved – and it would be.

Get Fit Time (20th July 1981)

The programme specifically designed for the thirty-eight year old executive was as follows:

- Pre-Stretch (5 minutes)
  - Head circle
  - Shoulder circle
  - Side stretch
  - Ankle stretch
  - Trunk twist
  - Thigh stretch
  - Hamstring and calf stretch
- Aerobic Activity
  - Motorised treadmill
    - Speed 3.5 m.p.h.
    - Duration 6 minutes

    Note: after 8 weeks 5 m.p.h. for 6 minutes
- Multigym

  The exercises on the multigym are intended for muscle endurance and not power (i.e. muscle building).

Weight kilos		Repetitions
50	Leg Press	10
30	Pull down	10
5	Bicep curl	10
	Dips	10
10	Hamstring curl	10

Weight kilos		Repetitions
20	Shoulder press	10
25	Bench press	10
–	Inclined sit-up	3
10	Wrist rolling	2
15	Leg extension	10

- Post-Stretch (Warm-down)

  The following activities are designed to wind you down and should therefore be carried out at lower stress levels.

  Static cycle 15 minutes (minimal resistance)

  Varying routine on a daily basis chosen from:
  - Step-ups
  - Punch ball
  - Rowing
  - Walking

The above programme was carefully monitored on a daily basis. Gradually the supervisor increased the aerobic and multigym activities as the cardio-vascular efficiency improved and weight began to fall. The charts summarising the results after an eight week period and after a year of starting the programme are indicated below.

As you will observe the results are quite dramatic in their improvement for the five categories chosen for demonstration purposes.

38 YEAR OLD MALE EXECUTIVE COMPARISON OF CARDIO VASCULAR AND WEIGHT FOR EIGHT WEEKS AND ONE YEAR AFTER PROGRAMME START

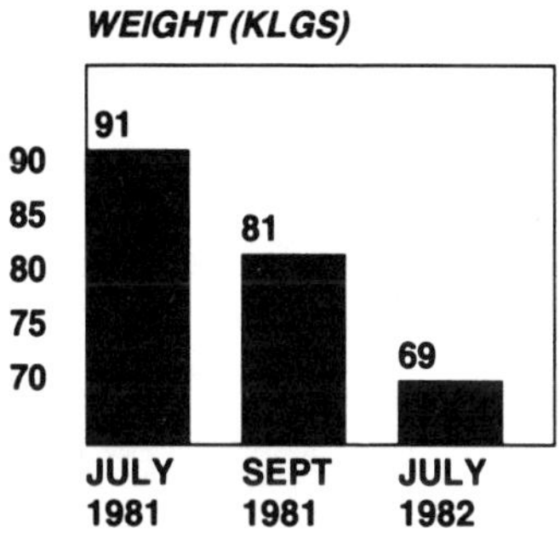

TABLE 13

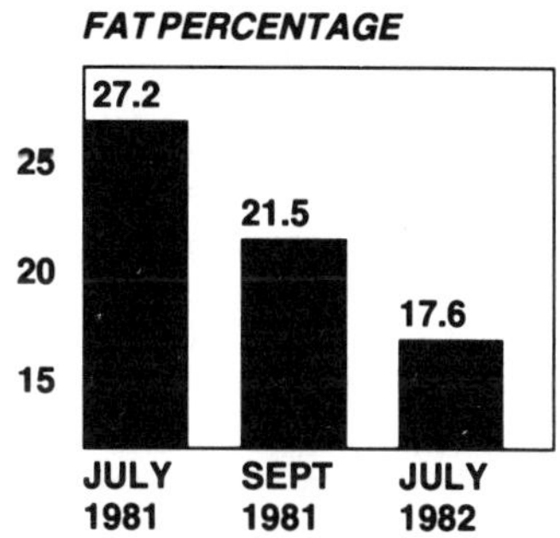

TABLE 14

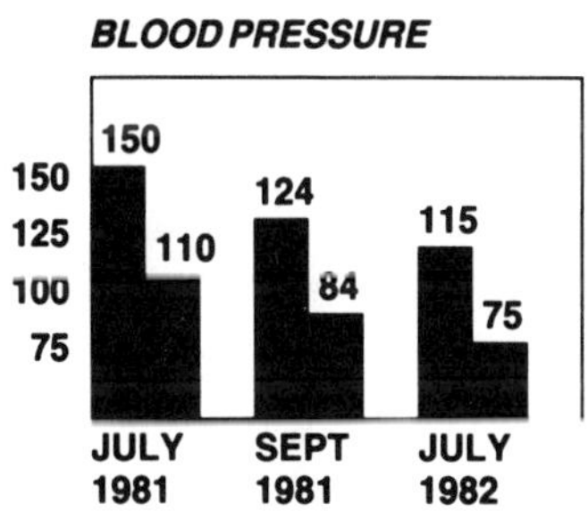

TABLE 15

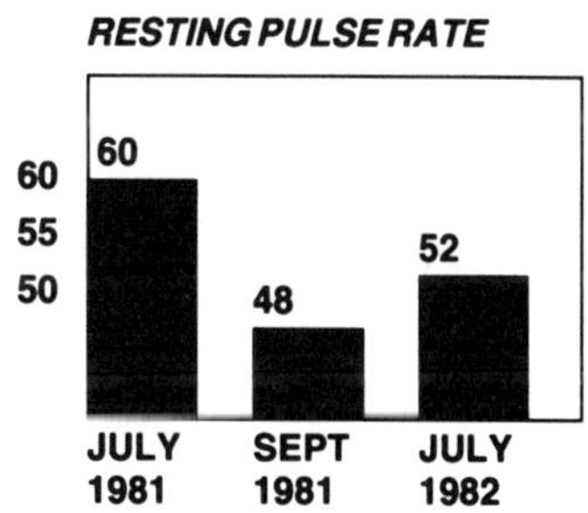

TABLE 16

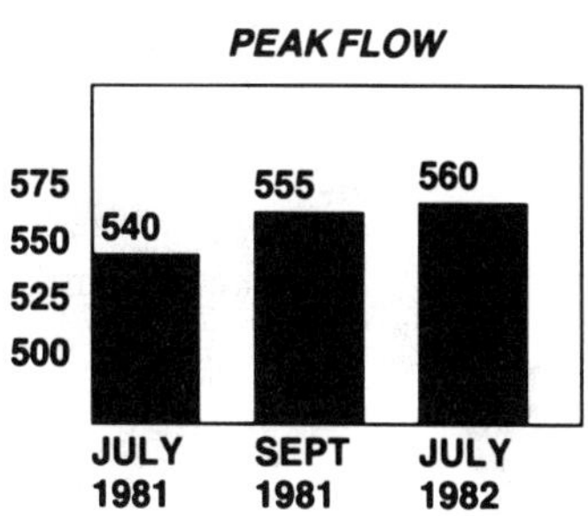

TABLE 17

It should be emphasised that these results are fairly representative and not an isolated case, provided that the recommended balance between diet and exercise is maintained. The executive looks good, feels good and follows a daily routine that he enjoys. Furthermore, he manages to keep this programme going despite an extremely demanding travel schedule (30% annually). After the hard work and dedication he really does consider it FUN, at least, most of the time.

Case 2. The programme followed by the forty one year old female executive was the same in structure as that for the thirty eight year old man. However, the one significant difference was that the aerobic activity was not on the motorised treadmill but on a static cycle. Running on the treadmill only began twelve weeks after the start of the programme. This was by personal choice, the result proved much the same.

The activities were very similar:

- Pre-stretch (as for man)
  - Aerobic
    - static cycle resistance 1
    - 25 kilometres per hour for 6 minutes

    Note: after 8 weeks 30 kilometres per hour for 20 minutes

- A circuit was devised which included 10 repetitions of the following:

– Sit-ups	– Bench jumps
– Rotations	– Dips
Modified	
– Press-ups	– Jack knife
– Squat thrusts	– Tuck jumps

Each exercise after 10 repetitions was interspersed with interval shuttle runs* around the gymnasium at a slow comfortable pace.

Again one can see from the following charts that the results are quite dramatic.

**A shuttle run means running backwards and forwards over the same ground.*

41 YEAR OLD FEMALE EXECUTIVE COMPARISON OF CARDIO VASCULAR AND WEIGHT FOR EIGHT WEEKS AND ONE YEAR AFTER FITNESS PROGRAMME START

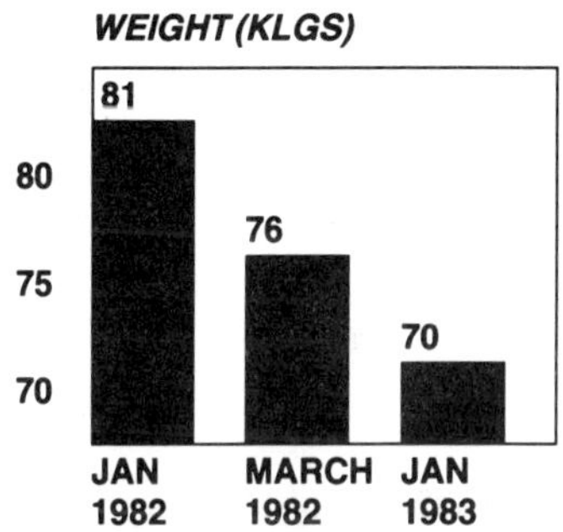

TABLE 18

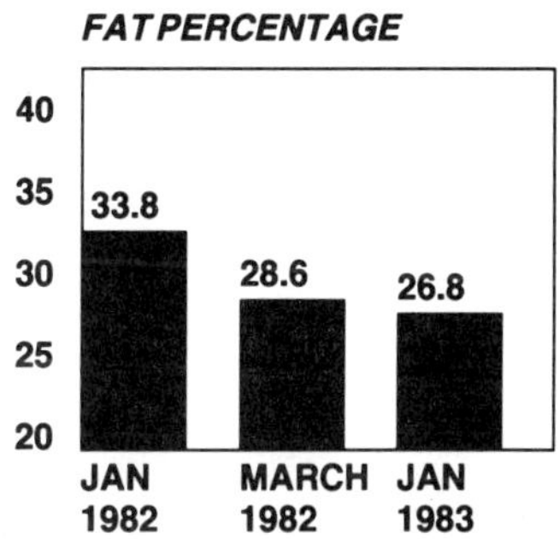

TABLE 19

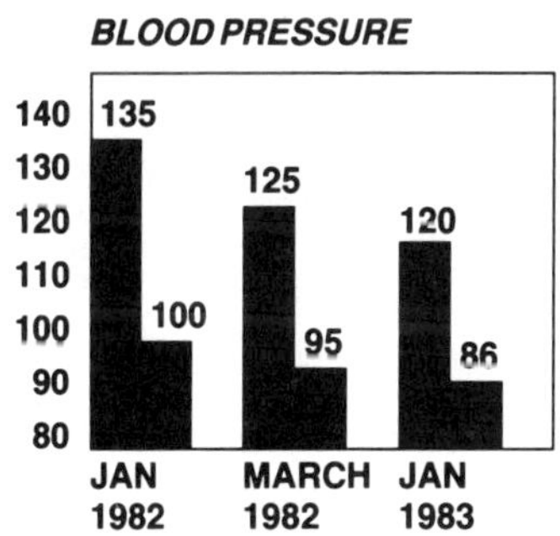

TABLE 20

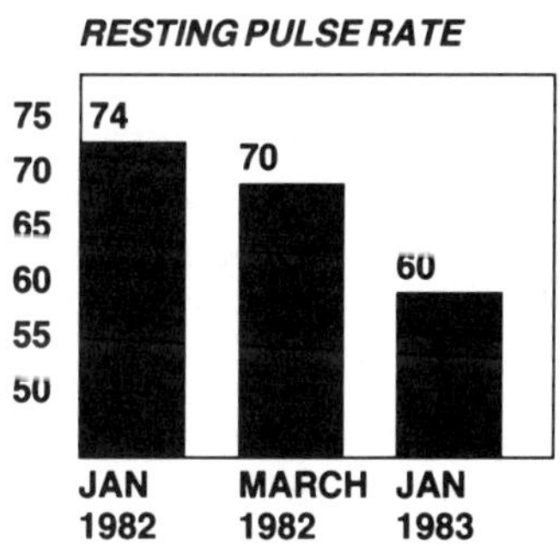

TABLE 21

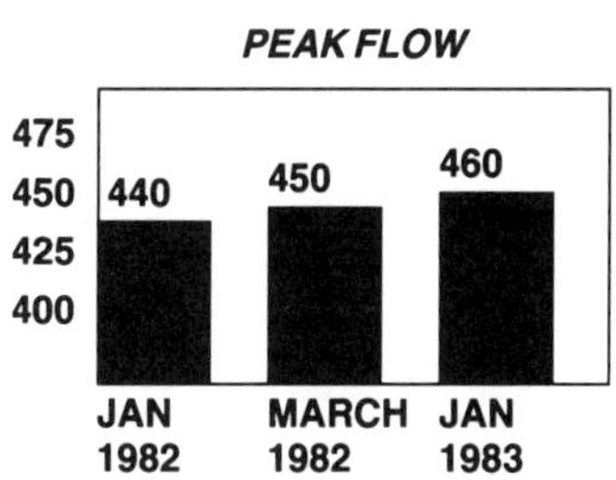

TABLE 22

VII

How can the Company help

The individual can go it alone. Many may decide to do just that. On the other hand, there is a growing awareness amongst the more enlightened companies that the executive lifestyle and demands on executives can be both stressful and sometimes counterproductive.

If days lost through illness can be reduced, performance increased and morale boosted, there is a desperate need to probe further.

The results of annual health screening are clearly visible and available to companies. The dramatic change in those results when a company professionally launches and backs up a company fitness programme are also available.

What steps should be taken to set up an executive fitness facility?

First, it is essential to have the endorsement of the company leaders. In addition, it is necessary to have an active sponsor who will support the programme.

Second, the company must decide to appoint qualified professional and support staff to set up and run the programme.

Third, participation of both men and women must be on a voluntary basis.

Fourth, the company must provide:

- Adequate floor space
- Equipment – treadmills
  static cycles
  weights (multi-gym)
- Changing rooms, lockers, showers and toilets
- Kit, including shorts, socks, vests and towels with daily laundry service, is a desirable extra

All the facilities should be designed to accommodate both men and women.

The experience of a number of companies is that 45% to 50% of the executives participate, with 35% to 40% attending regularly.

The company can go further by providing sauna or jacuzzi facilities or perhaps a swimming pool. These added advantages may be funded by the Sports and Social Club, which is a natural extension of the fitness programme.

Other desirable spin-offs could include:

- Outward-Bound courses
- Competitive events
  - Fun runs
  - Marathons
  - In-house superstars
  - Best performance within age group etc

The idea behind augmenting the general fitness programme is to enhance self motivation and get competitive spirit injected into the programme.

Executives normally thrive on competition and it is with this in mind that added dimensions to the programme make it all the more interesting.

The company can support individuals who achieve pre-determined benchmarks (say a T shirt for 1000 miles running). A medal, certificate or a cup for the best performance. Recognition of achievement in the company magazine – there are many and various ways of keeping the interest alive.

The company can also sponsor events such as fun runs and marathons, which makes the employees feel genuinely involved.

To give some idea of size and cost the following may prove to be useful guidelines when exploring the prospect of establishing a fitness centre:

Space requirements: A 3000 sq.ft. facility will accommodate 10 to 12 persons at one time. Lockers and showers will need additional space. Don't forget male and female requirements in the design!

Cost: This depends on the quality of product and the degree of sophistication needed. Basic equipment should not exceed £10,000. Conversion costs of existing facilities could be in the region of £20–£25,000.

Some companies share the facilities, which has a number of benefits – including assistance with defining the costs. Saunas, solaria, rest rooms, jacuzzi are the icing on the cake. Although not essential they often have a morale-boosting effect.

In addition to the one time cost there are the day-to-day operating costs, of which 80% are salaries and wages; the other 20% being made up of heating and lighting together with laundry costs of kit and towels. Toiletries also feature in the package.

Benefit analysis: A careful analysis over a three-year period has indicated a marked reduction in lost days. The target to aim for is for every £1 expended £3 will be recouped by less days taken off through illness.

Naturally, the intangible benefits are much greater:

- Improved productivity through greater energy
- Increased morale as a result of individual and group motivation
- Greater loyalty to the caring company.
- Competing with one's peers, employees and bosses in a different environment.
- Extended life expectancy.

It really is worthwhile.

VIII

'Crossroads'

The book has concentrated on getting people to a general level of fitness. If you have followed the exercise programme carefully and been moderate in your eating and drinking habits then you will be approaching 'par' within 8 to 12 weeks.

You have arrived at the 'Crossroads'. Where do you go from here?

1. Stop
2. Continue an expanded programme
3. Pursue your favourite recreation activity
4. Specialise in a particular sport
5. Go in for martial arts

1. The decision to stop the programme entirely could be a very difficult one. Unless of course you have sustained a particular injury. The daily routine will be established; family, group and peer pressure will make stopping a problem. It is amazing how quickly the benefits of an 8–12 week fitness programme are eroded once the daily routine is stopped and you revert to the indolent lifestyle.

   It is time to stop and pause. Just recapitulate on the motivational pros and cons, think again about the ideas and thoughts addressed during the build-up to the programme. What about the rest of the group and how do they feel about quitting?

It is interesting to note that the drop-out percentage on the authors' course is around 5%. Individuals who modify the programme by relaxing the daily schedule to a more leisurely pace make up another, say, 5%. What happens to the other 90%? These fall into the categories 2 to 5.

2. Continue an expanded programme.

   To date the programme has been relatively simple. Wider dimensions can be added through:

   - a gymnasium
   - specific training
     - interval training
     - Fartlck training
     - weight training

The Gymnasium

Most areas nowadays have a leisure centre where there are gymnasia with up-to-date apparatus. Often these are supervised by physical educationists. But in some instances, although the apparatus is available, people are left to work out their own programme. This chapter will help those who may not be too sure of how to use the apparatus or indeed how to formulate their work-out. First of all, we will look at the small exercise room that may only contain the barest essentials. An exercise bicycle, rowing machine, skipping ropes, and some loose weights with bar-bells. This may be in the local football or rugby club or it may even form your own 'garage gym'.

Pre-Stretch

Since you will already be aware of your pre-stretch exercises there is no further need to discuss this, but of course these will be 'part one' of any fitness programme.

Aerobics using the static cycle

Reference to the cycle ergometer fitness index, page 65 will indicate your level of work rate using the exercise bicycle. Remember that the resistance setting on the machine is best set at a level that closely approximates to road cycling, in other words, sufficient friction to necessitate effort but not strain. We are not using the bicycle to build-up leg power, so whatever the reason for discontinuing, it should not be one of localised fatigue in the leg muscles. Having achieved the final stage on the cycle ergometer fitness index, further progression may be made by increasing speed and distance. For example, a good work-out for a fit man of forty years of age, may be 12.8 kilometres at a speed of 32 kilometres per hour, this will take 24 minutes.

Rowing Machine

If one chooses to use the rowing machine for aerobic benefit, once again resistance should be set at a low level. It is difficult to compare work loads in comparison to the bicycle, because the overall muscle work in rowing is much greater, but based on the consumption of oxygen for each method, the following table will provide a close guide. Remember that most of the muscle work involved in rowing should come from the legs, the arms only being bent at the end of each stroke.

ROWING MACHINE INDEX

AGE	20-30	30-40	40-45	45-50	50-55	55-60	WEEK
Strokes per minute	24	24	24	22	22	20	1
DURATION	5.30m	5.0m	4.30m	4.0m	3.30m	3.0m	
Strokes per minute	24	24	24	22	22	20	2
DURATION	6.0m	5.30m	5.0m	4.30m	4.0m	3.30m	
Strokes per minute	26	26	24	24	22	20	3
DURATION	6.30m	6.0m	5.30m	5.0m	4.30m	4.0m	
Strokes per minute	28	28	26	24	22	20	4
DURATION	7.0m	6.30m	6.0m	5.30m	5.0m	4.30m	
Strokes per minute	28	28	28	26	24	22	5
DURATION	7.30m	7.0m	6.0m	6.0m	5.30m	5.0m	
Strokes per minute	30	30	28	26	24	22	6
DURATION	8.0m	7.30m	7.0m	6.30m	6.0m	5.30m	

Progress by moving to a lower age category for each succeeding week.

TABLE 23

Step Ups

The performance of step-ups to achieve aerobic benefit is not generally as acceptable or successful as running, cycling, swimming or rowing. This is because local fatigue in the leg muscles occurs before the work has been performed long enough to provide cardio-vascular benefit. However, with sufficient practice the leg muscles will eventually become accustomed to the work, so that periods long enough for training benefit will be achieved. Reference to the Fitness Assessment Ready Reckoner will explain how to perform the step-ups and the table below will provide a guide to progression.

STEP-UP INDEX

AGE	*20-30*	*30-40*	*40-45*	*45-50*	*50-55*	*55-60*	*WEEK*
No. of Step Ups	72	72	60	60	48	36	1
TIME	3.0m	3.0m	2.30m	2.30m	2.0m	1.30m	
No. of Step Ups	84	72	72	60	60	48	2
TIME	3.30m	3.0m	3.0m	2.30m	2.30m	2.0m	
No. of Step Ups	98	84	72	72	60	60	3
TIME	4.0m	3.30m	3.0m	3.0m	2.30m	2.30m	
No. of Step Ups	114	98	84	72	72	60	4
TIME	4.30m	4.0m	3.30m	3.0m	3.0m	2.30m	
No. of Step Ups	132	114	98	84	72	72	5
TIME	5.0m	4.30m	4.0m	3.30m	3.0m	3.0m	
No. of Step Ups	152	132	114	98	84	72	6
TIME	5.30m	5.0m	4.30m	4.0m	3.30m	3.0m	

Progress by moving to a lower age category for each succeeding week.

TABLE 24

The comparatively slow build-up is designed to accustom the leg muscles to the work-load. Because of this, once the performer has achieved the final target as shown for week six in the twenty to thirty age group, he should then progress by increasing the number of step-ups, keeping at the same rate, and adding 30 seconds per week. The ultimate duration of the step-up work-out should not exceed 15 minutes. To progress beyond this time may result in over-use injury occurring to the joints and soft tissues of the legs.

Skipping

Skipping with ropes involves a certain degree of skill, agility and co-ordination, so it does not find very wide favour as a means of achieving aerobic benefit. However, once the skill has been mastered skipping is a useful method of training for cardio-vascular endurance. Fatigue levels are reached very quickly so a lot of practice and training is necessary before one is able to sustain the effort for long enough periods. Therefore it will be seen that progression is rather slow and so graduation occurs automatically. Skipping can be very usefully employed in your fitness programme by using interval training methods. See page 150.

Musculo-Skeletal

Once having completed the aerobic part of your work-out, the loose weights will provide the means for musculo-skeletal exercise. The minimum requirement for this is one barbell and dumbell kit, consisting of one long bar with collars plus two 5 kg weight discs and one short bar with collars plus two 2.5 kg weight discs. Your weight training schedule should be designed to provide an all-round muscular toning programme. The basic exercises for this are illustrated. It is recommended that repetitions do not exceed ten for each exercise, but the number of sets should depend upon one's level of fitness. It is not always possible for an unfit person to complete a circuit.

For definition purposes the following will apply:
Exercises × 10 repetitions = 1 set
All exercises (4 have been explained) × 10 repetitions = 4 sets. 4 sets = 1 circuit.

Those persons who may be unused to heavy muscular work should start out using only the lighter weight discs. Don't forget to do some abdominal work as illustrated – pages 89/90.

Exercise 1: Bicep Curls

FIGURE 53

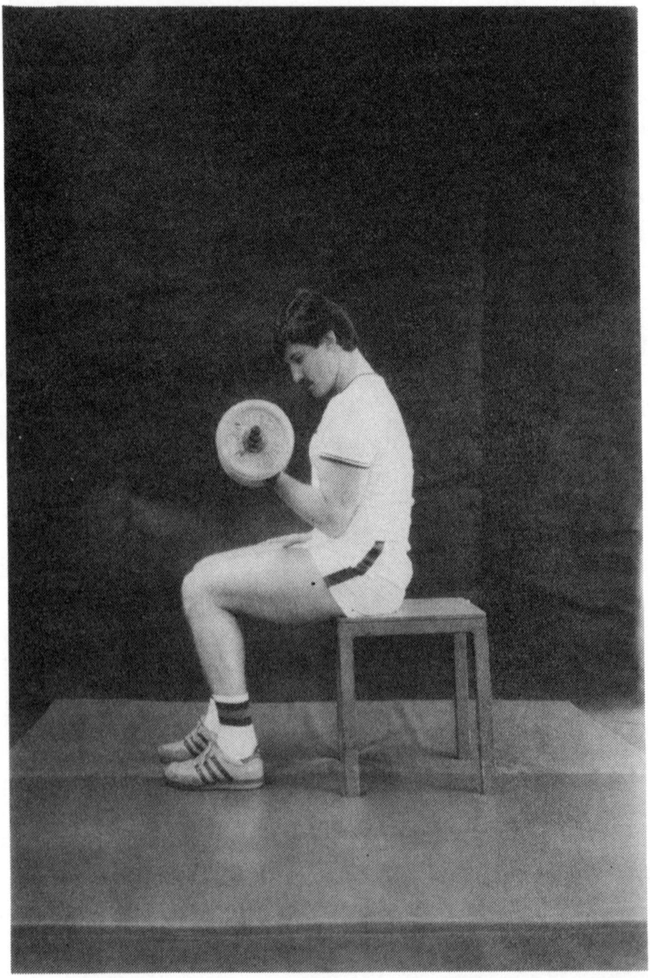

Exercise 2: Shoulder Press

FIGURE 54

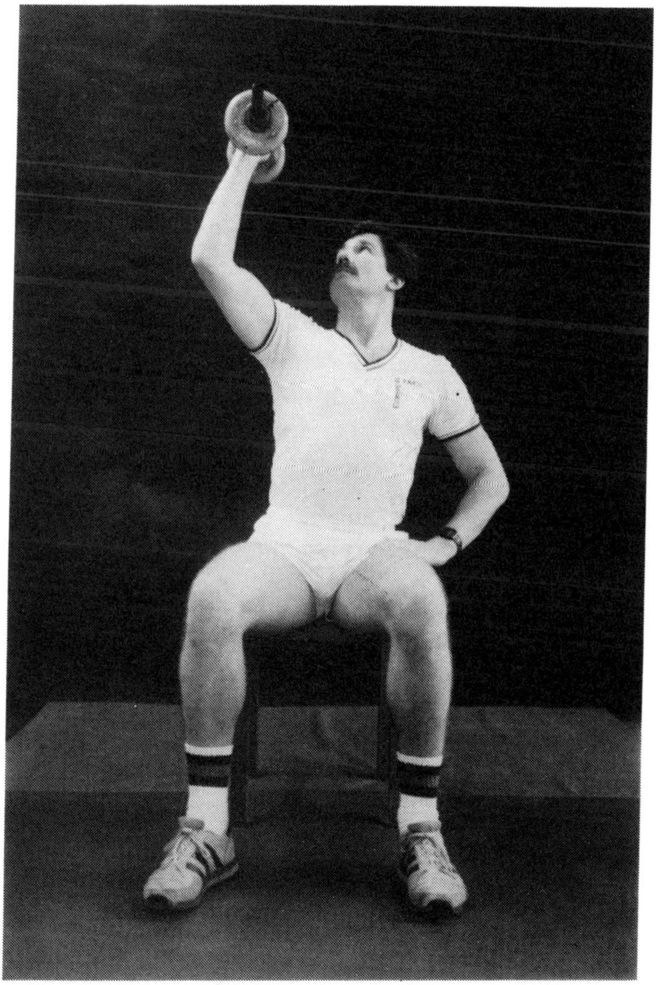

Exercise 3: Deltoid Lift

FIGURE 55

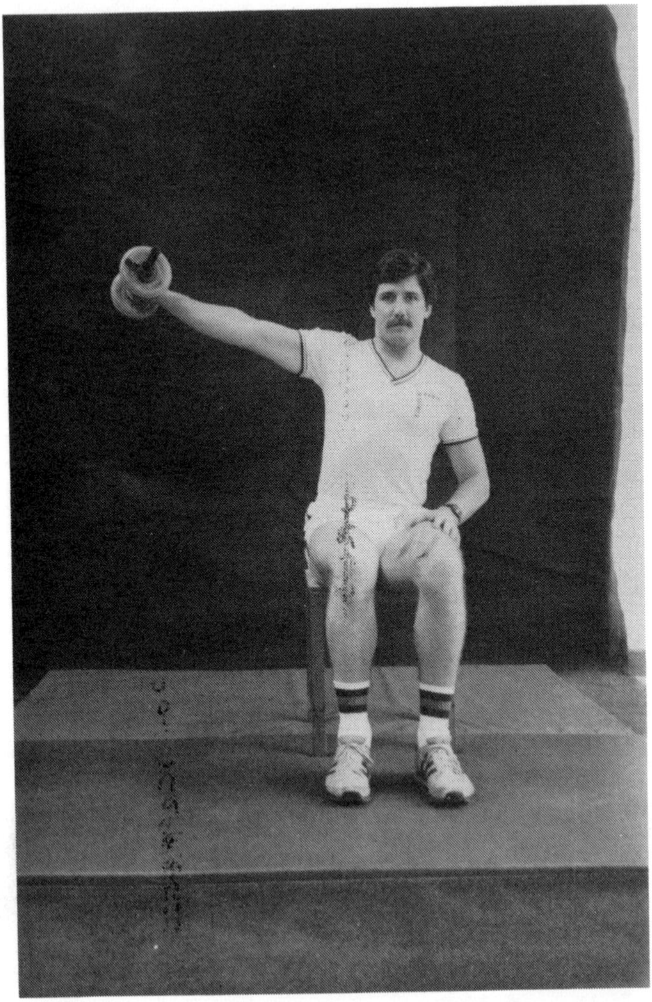

Exercise 4: Forearm Twist

FIGURE 56

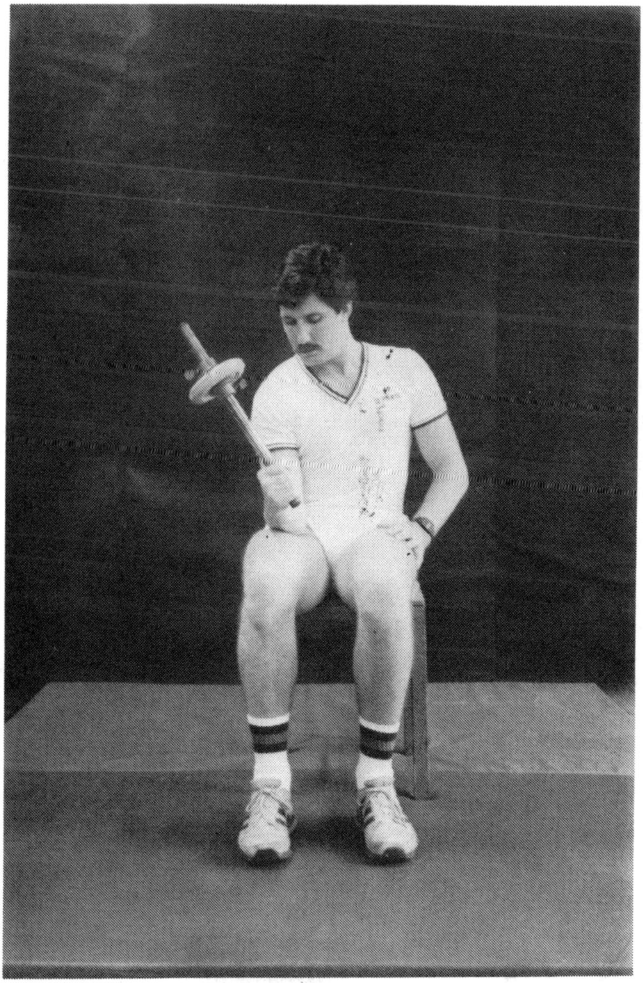

Exercise 5: Chest Press

FIGURE 57

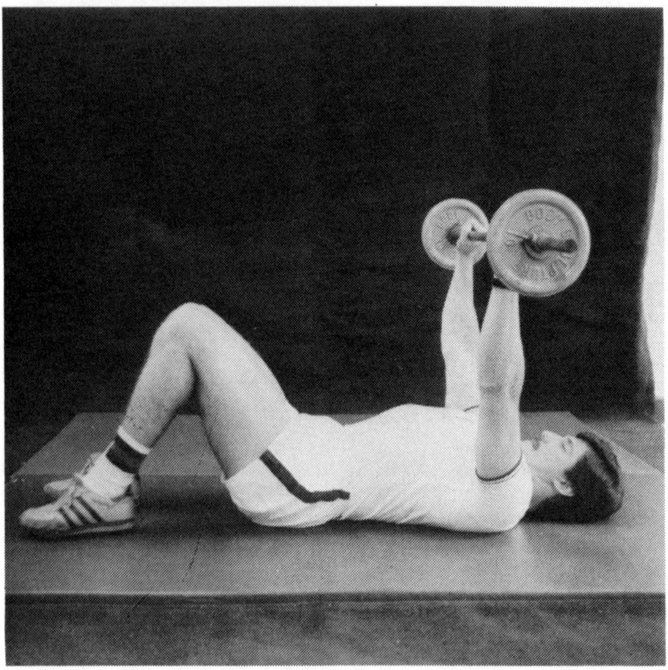

Exercise 6: Half Squats

FIGURE 58

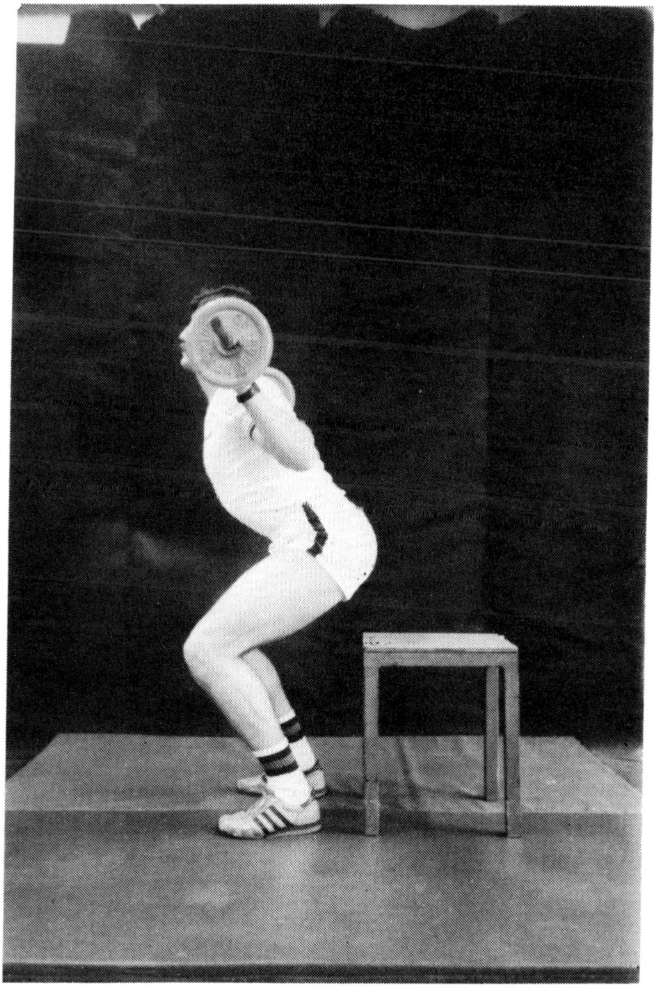

GENERAL CHARACTERISTICS OF COMMONLY USED TREADMILL PROTOCOLS

Protocol	*No. of Stages*	*Range of Speed (mph)*	*Range of Grade (%)*	*Duration (Minutes/ Stages)*	*Total Time Elapsed (Min)*	*Observation*	*Pulse Rate Pre Post Exercises*	
BRUCE	7	1.7–6.0	10–22	3	21	Applicable for moderately fit persons up to stage 4. After stage 4, trained men and athletes.	66	180
BALKE	22	3.3	2–22	1	22	Applicable for trained women and moderately fit men. Because of the slow build-up of the incline, the workload isn't noticeable until Grade 16%. The calfs were put under strain and discomfort was felt for some time following exercises	68	178
NAUGHTON	13	1.0–2.0	0–22	2	30	Applicable for Women, Patients on rehabilitation. Strenuous after grade 15%.	65	130
ELLESTAD	4	1.7–5.0	10	2–3	10	Applicable for cardiac rehabilitation. Men and women. This test could be managed by most, but the very unfit.	68	140
NATIONAL EXERCISE PROJECT	10	2.0–3.0	0–17.5	3	30	Applicable for male cardiac training and female fitness training. Calf pain and stiffness, a slow graduation.	66	144

TABLE 25

There are many more exercises that may readily come to mind, but we have confined this section to those exercises we consider most important. Remember to train not strain, lift weights by easy progressions, and make sure weight discs are secure on the bar.

Your whole work out should end up with the post stretch exercises as illustrated on pages 84/86.

The Complete Fitness Workshop

Modern gymnasia today usually possess the latest design in apparatus including running treadmills, computerised exercise bicycles, universal and comprehensive weight training units, and measuring equipment. Some companies may have in-house facilities and the best hotels usually provide a fitness room. One of the frequent problems, however, is lack of properly qualified staff, so that the apparatus tends to be used incorrectly. In this section we discuss the various methods of exercising using modern equipment.

The Running Treadmill – some motorised treadmills are designed to incorporate gradients of up to 25%, and these are useful in testing for cardio-vascular response to known work loads (Protocols). Otherwise, most motorised treadmills are quite sufficient for normal fitness programmes as their speed ranges are usually from 1 to 10 miles per hour.

Before using a treadmill, one should have undertaken a pulse recovery rate test as outlined in the Fitness Assessment Ready Reckoner – page 24. Any result below average in this test demands further training on a bicycle ergometer, unless speeds on the treadmill do not exceed walking pace. Reference to the table on jogging graduation page 63 will provide the necessary degrees of progression for the beginner. Some gymnasia with individualised programmes have qualified physical therapists or exercise physiologists in attendance. Very often, this results in progression by Protocol testing which is one of the best methods to evaluate necessary programme modification. Protocols are designs of measurement to evaluate fitness levels. They are generally used in treadmill and cycle ergometry testing. It may be worthwhile to discuss some of the better known protocols designed by some American physiologists, with comments on their measuring values. In researching this, five fit young men and one woman took part, and their comments were noted. A sample of their results have been calculated and a mean arrived at.

General Characteristics

There is no reason why specialists in physical education, and those involved in preventive medicine, should not design their own protocols to suit the particular levels of ability in which they may specialise. The Hughes–Sharp protocol shown below was designed by two Remedial Gymnasts who successfully found a formula that has a comprehensive cover for all levels. Furthermore, it is a protocol that equates very closely with corresponding work on a bicycle ergometer, see Table 27. Because of its slow graduation, the participants of the test do not need to 'warm-up', thus their starting pulse rates are not unduly raised.

Interval Training

This form of training is characterised by short rest periods between bursts of intense level exercise. In spite of the intervals of rest, the pulse rate is never allowed to fall back to pre-exercise levels. The principle is to gradually cut down the duration of the intervals while slowly building up the duration of exercise. In this way, exercise tolerance is improved as heart-rate recovery time lessens. The type of exercise activity

HUGHES-SHARP PROTOCOL

This protocol is performed for a maximum of 15 minutes at a constant elevation of 10%. There are also a maximum 10 stages, each lasting 1.5 minutes. Each stage increases in speed by 0.5 miles per hour (0.8 Kilometres per hour).

STAGE	*MPH*	*KPH*
1	2.0	3.2
2	2.5	4.0
3	3.0	4.8
4	3.5	5.6
5	4.0	6.4
6	4.5	7.2
7	5.0	8.0
8	5.5	8.8
9	6.0	9.6
10	6.5	10.4

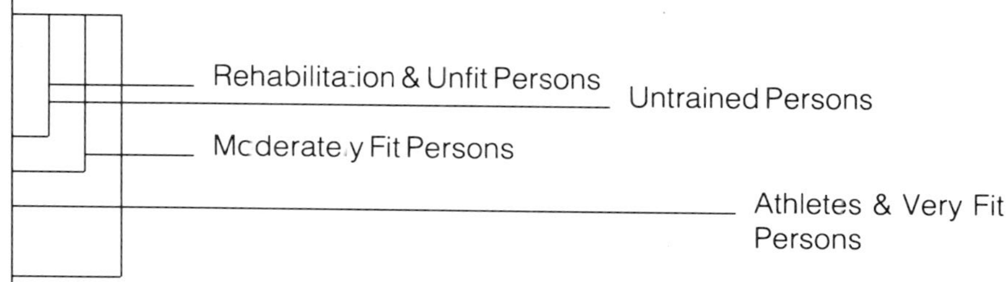

TABLE 26

PERFORMANCE COMPARISON BETWEEN
20wts per min = 0.3 VO per min.

'MONARCH' CYCLE @ 30 KPH.	WATTS	'TREADMILL' @ 10% elev.
¼	20	3.2 KPH
½	40	4 KPH
¾	60	4.8 KPH
1	80	5.6 KPH
1¼	100	6.4 KPH
1½	120	7.2 KPH
1¾	140	8.0 KPH
2	160	8.8 KPH
2¼	180	9.2 KPH
2½	200	10.2 KPH

TABLE 27

RESISTANCE

that is chosen will depend on the desired result. The squash player for example rarely has spells of high activity for longer than a minute at a time. Accordingly his chosen exercise should be explosive in nature with short intervals. On the other hand the middle distance runner may require longer periods of activity interspersed with sharp sprints and longer periods of rest.

Skipping has already been mentioned as an excellent form of exercise for interval training. An example of how one's programme can be devised, using this activity, is set out. Using alternate leg skipping without rebound, skip at a rate of approximately 150 jumps per minute with 15 seconds rest for the first stint. This will raise the heart rate sufficiently high to form the platform for the remainder of your work-out. As the work-out continues, slow down your skipping rate keeping the 15 second rests. When the skipping rate drops below 100, change to double take-off skipping with rebounds, cutting down the rest periods to 10 seconds. Eventually cut out all rest periods until skipping is continuous for as long as possible.

Cycling is a very sound alternative to jogging for aerobic exercise, and in many cases is preferred especially by those who would rather work-out at home. The static cycle lends itself very well to interval training of progressive intensity and will produce positive effects on the cardio-vascular system. It must also be considered as a safe method of continued training, during periods when perhaps jogging is contra-indicated. It is known that the stresses imposed on the ankle, knee and hip joints in cycling are much less than those caused by jogging. The elderly, the obese, and the sedentary person starting out on an exercise programme may do well to use the static cycle as an alternative to jogging. One of the disadvantages, once the individual has attained a reasonably high level of fitness, is boredom.

Some of this boredom may be relieved by incorporating interval training. The procedure adopted will depend upon the subject's age, fitness level, and to some extent leg power. But the following method has been used with a great deal of success with subjects of both sexes aged between thirty-five and forty-five.

The bicycle used was a Monark standard type ergometer, but most static bicycles equipped with a fly-wheel and belt friction device can be regulated to suit the procedure.

Stage 1 The subjects should start by warming-up for three minutes at a low friction resistance and at approximately 65-75 revolutions per minute (r.p.m.).

Stage 2 This is then followed up by increasing the resistance to medium intensity, whilst maintaining the r.p.m. at 90. The duration of this period ceases only when the r.p.m. falls below 90 for more than 5 seconds.

Stage 3 A rest is then allowed. This rest period should be long enough to allow the pulse rate to fall by a third. For example, if 150 beats per minute is recorded at the end of stage 2, then stage 4 should not commence until the heart beats per minute fall below 100 (repeat for stage 5).

Stage 4 The next burst consists of an increase of r.p.m. to 100 dropping the resistance to low friction, again this period is carried out for three minutes.

Stage 5 Another burst of activity at 90 r.p.m. but keeping up the pedal rate until it drops for 5 seconds, and once again resting to allow a third of exercise pulse-rate recovery, before starting again at stage 2.

Progression may be made by increasing the work periods or decreasing the rest periods. This work-out should be performed at least four times weekly. The ultimate target of work-out duration should be in excess of 20 minutes.

Using the above examples, most individuals would

find it not too difficult to design their own format for interval training in whatever activities they choose.

Fartlek Training

This is a form of training which combines variable speed running with stints of calisthenics. It can be extremely demanding and is excellent training for those individuals who have reached a high level of fitness, and wish to progress even further. This type of training was first developed by a Swedish athletics coach called Gosta Holmer who was concerned about the boredom of long distance running and its effect on the athletes. Its principles lie in variation and getting away from the humdrum track or road forms of training. The first essential therefore is to find a park or open country with changes in terrain and which is accessible to the public. In some communities with leisure centres special trails have been laid out specifically for Fartlek training. It is fortunate that in most areas of Great Britain one does not have far to go to find a suitable piece of open ground, where one may design one's own course. But even if one has to use roads and pavements, there is usually ample opportunity to use the associated structures in designing one's training course. In many ways Fartlek training amounts to interval workouts performed in open areas. The design of a course should incorporate short flat stretches for sprinting, longer undulating terrain for slower running, and stations for calisthenic exercises interpersed at intervals around the whole course.

For those individuals who are in training for competitive events or team games, Fartlek courses offer the chance to simulate the competition by the inclusion of specific activity. For example, the football player could introduce a ball to control as he negotiates the course, using the lower twigs of tree branches for heading practice on the run. The sprinter could incorporate mock starting blocks created by carefully placed rocks at intervals. And working in pairs, rugby players could practise ball passing on the route. There is tremendous scope for all kinds of variation, without using costly apparatus, and some companies that may be fortunate to have their own areas of open ground should consider the planning of a permanent course that could be used by their employees. Of course there is another factor which must be considered in Fartlek training and that is the weather and changing seasons.

The winter is perhaps the season that demands more imagination in constructing the course or in the use of an existing trail. In snowy conditions skis may be put to good use for cross-country, without detracting from the degree of effort involved. Muddy conditions are probably the worst, because using the course will not only aggravate matters but could prove dangerous. The course distance should, if possible, take up to at least 40 minutes to complete, and courses of ten miles are not unusual. In smaller areas it may be necessary for participants to complete the course several times to achieve a good workout.

As has been said, the construction of the course depends on the type of training required, and the imagination of the athletes in its use. Some examples are here set out; they include one for athletes, one for squash players, and one for general fitness maintenance.

The participant may take the course in a casual light-hearted way, or pressurise himself to improve his performance. Whatever the approach, it should be fun, the word 'Fartlek' roughly translated means 'Speedplay'.

Athletes course Distance 5 miles 15 stations

1. Pre-stretch exercises
2. Jog 1 mile
3. Sprint 100 yards
4. Medium pace run ½ mile
5. 20 sit ups
6. Medium pace run 1 mile
7. Sprint 60 yards
8. 20 squat thrusts
9. Medium pace run 1½ miles
10. 20 press-ups (with rests if necessary)
11. Sprint 60 yards
12. Jog ½ mile
13. 20 Tuck jumps
14. Use up remaining energy running 'home'
15. Post-stretch exercises.

Squash Players Course 2 miles 12 stations

1. Pre-stretch exercises
2. Jog 1 mile
3. 20 short shuttle runs (10 yards)
4. Jog ½ mile
5. 20 sit-ups
6. Sprint 60 yards
7. 20 single leg squats
8. 20 short shuttle runs touching ground with hands at end of each shuttle (10 yards)
9. Jog 600 yards
10. 20 press-ups (resting if necessary)
11. Use up remaining energy running 'home'
12. Post-stretch exercises

General Fitness Course 4 miles 11 stations

1. Pre-stretch exercises
2. Jog 1 mile
3. Step-ups (25 each leg)
4. Jog 1 mile
5. 25 sit-ups
6. Sprint 60 yards
7. Jog 1 mile
8. 25 press-ups (resting if necessary)
9. Sprint 60 yards
10. Jog home
11. Post-stretch exercises

Now get out and have fun

Weight Training

Exercise to gain strength, muscle endurance, or to improve physique is probably best performed with weight resistance. In previous chapters it has been shown that one's own body-weight can be utilised in this way if apparatus is unavailable. However, the up-to-date gymnasium will probably have one of the many comprehensive weight systems, such as the Multi-gym. These consist of several 'stations' forming an integral part of the whole unit. Weight resistance is set on each station very easily by inserting a steel pin into the appropriate socket. But whatever the form of weight resistance, the principles of training are the same. First one should indentify one's requirements. Do you need a strength programme? Do you just wish to maintain muscle tone and endurance? Or do you want to combine the latter with circuits so that some aerobic benefit is achieved?

It should be understood that most weight-training programmes are of an anaerobic nature, like many other activities that have rest periods or fluctuations in pulse-rate intensity. This is because the level of oxygen demanded by the activity is more than the cardio-vascular system can supply. This leads to an oxygen debt and a build up of lactic acid, which limits high activity periods, demanding cessation, or a slowing down of intensity levels. It will be seen by the following tables how one may, by adjusting weight resistance and speed performance, select the programme best suited to one's needs.

Training for Strength using the Multi-Gym System

Procedure

1. Measure the maximum weight at which you are able to overcome inertia, this does not mean performing a full movement, but that you are able to initiate a movement of resistance.

2. Now select a resistance of at least 5 kg but not more than 10 kg less than the maximum.

3. Carry out at least three repetitions at each station resting for 2 minutes between the stations.

4. Repeat the circuit at least three times.

5. Record your performance and adjust when necessary.

Training for Muscle Endurance and Tone using the Multi-Gym System

Procedure

1. As for strength programme.

2. Select the resistance of half that of maximum, favouring the higher figure if exactly half is not possible.

3. Carry out and record the maximum number of repetitions possible at each station, taking as much rest as necessary between the stations. The repetitions should be performed with only enough pause to separate one from the other.

4. Stations that work on body weight resistance, such as chinning and sit-ups are also carried out to maximum.

5. A gradual build-up of repetitions should be aimed at until re-adjustment of the measure of (1) above is necessary. Then continue as from (2) above.

Training for Tone with Aerobic Benefit using the Multi-Gym System

Procedure

1. As for (1) in previous tables.
2. Select a resistance of at least 5 kg but not more than 10 kg below the weights for muscle endurance.
3. Perform at least ten but not more than fifteen repetitions at each station as fast as possible without cheating, no resting between stations.
4. Stations that work on body-weight resistance are performed for a third of maximum.
5. Perform at least three circuits in as fast a time as possible. Check pulse-rate.
6. Record total time; on subsequent sessions attempt to cut total time. When this is no longer possible increase circuits by one.

In all these examples, one's natural ceiling of ability will determine one's progress.

3. & 4. Pursuing a favourite recreation or sport

The fitness programme of getting up to 'par' and continuing beyond has concentrated on the four key aspects of aerobics, obesity, power (strength) and flexibility. Some people want to keep fit and look good merely to do a worthwhile job in the garden at week-ends, keep up with the kids or to get the best from their favourite recreational activity.

Having got to a reasonable level of fitness you may want to understand how this complements your recreational activities. Naturally, the recreational sport to be pursued often depends on age, sex, work or family environment, friends and personal choice as much as health status. It is almost certain, however, that participation in the health programme will extend horizons.

Having referred to body types and how they influence 'preferences' it is quite obvious that a professional adviser will guide people towards their strengths. For example, a person who is a keen runner need not stop exercising if there is a minor injury (such as a blister, or minor foot or knee ailment). He or she may be encouraged to swim or to use the static cycle.

How can they measure the equal activity level in each of the sports?

The following table will enable you to assess what benefit you get from the sport you pursue and how it fits in with the training programme.

It is considered worthwhile to say a few words about seven recreational sporting activities. These have been selected because of their benefit to weight loss, power, flexibility and aerobic endurance. The seven selected from the following table are:

- Cycling
- Dancing
- Golf
- Swimming
- Judo (see below)
- Rowing
- Squash

BENEFITS

		Calorie Expenditure per hour	*Aerobic Benefit*	*Fat Loss*	*Power*	*Flexibility*
1.	BADMINTON (Competitive)	480	M	M	L	M
2.	CANOEING	750	M	M	H	L
3.	CRICKET	250				
	BATTING		L	L	M	H
	BOWLING	450				
4.	CYCLING (Hard)	600	M	H	L	H
5.	DANCING (Disco)	250	M	H	L	H
6.	FOOTBALL	350/500	M	H	M	H
7.	GOLF	300	L	L	L	M
8.	GYMNASTICS	500	M	H	H	H
9.	WALKING	480/600				
	UPHILL		H	M	L	L
	UPSTAIRS	600/800				
10.	JOGGING	600	H	H	M	L
11.	JUDO	750	L	M	H	H
12.	ROWING	840	H	H	H	M
13.	SAILING	500	L	L	M	L
14.	SQUASH	700	M	M	M	H
15.	SWIMMING (Hard)	650	H	M	M	M
16.	TENNIS	500	M	M	M	H
17	WEIGHT LIFTING	500	L	L	H	L

Key: L = low; M = medium; H = high.

TABLE 28

In addition to the above, reference will be made to orienteering and martial arts in conjunction with judo.

Cycling

This has many advantages as a form of exercise for it costs little after the initial purchase of a suitable machine, its use as a mode of travel is cheap, interesting and convenient. For individuals who dislike jogging or for those who are prone to impact injury through running on hard or uneven surfaces, this form of activity provides an excellent alternative. In order to achieve aerobic benefit from cycling one needs to maintain a steady speed of around fifteen miles per hour for at least twenty minutes.

If you are interested in track racing or cycle touring it is possible to receive coaching from experts by joining one of the many clubs situated all over the country. Another form of sport that may appeal to enthusiasts of cycling is Cyclo-Cross which is a combination of cross country cycling and cross country running. This is a competitive sport which requires a high degree of fitness and strength. Sometimes carrying the bicycle over rough terrain and in order to negotiate certain obstacles, can be very fatiguing.

For further information contact:

The British Cycling Federation,
16 Upper Woburn Place,
London, WC1H 0QC.

or

The British Cyclo-Cross Association,
8 Bellam Road,
Hampton Magna,
Warwicks.

Folk Dancing

Any person who has had the pleasure of watching Morris dancers performing will have not failed to notice the high level of fitness required. The English Folk Dance and Song Society together with The Morris Ring have a repertoire of some four hundred country dances. Membership is open to all age groups and there are clubs all over the country. As well as offering the opportunity of keeping fit the social aspect is an important element that can be enjoyed by the whole family as well as individuals. No special clothing is required for the usual get-togethers and dances, but during festivals, costume dances are often performed. These costumes can usually be made quite easily, most members make their own. The pleasures one may derive from the dancing, the social atmosphere and the exercise are complemented by the knowledge that one is helping to preserve our nation's heritage.

For further details contact:

The English Folk Dance and Song Society,
Cecil Sharp House,
2 Regents Park Road,
London, N.W.1.

Golf

Although as an activity golf is largely anaerobic, it is nevertheless good exercise to supplement one's fitness programme. It requires little strength, but a lot of flexibility from shoulders, hips and spine. As a rehabilitation activity for persons recovering from illness or other forms of disablement it is excellent. It can be played by both male and female and at almost any age. For the older executive who does not aspire to being super-fit but just wants to maintain his health and get some exercise, it is a sport that is highly recommended.

There are many municipal courses all over the country where one does not need to be a member, and where green fees are not exorbitant. But if one wants to join a club it is often difficult to become a member straight away, and sometimes the fees are very high.

Equipment initially, can be very expensive, but afterwards, running costs can be cut down to the purchase of golf balls and small items to be replaced.

For further information contact the:

English Golf Union,
12a Denmark Street,
Wokingham,
Berkshire, RG11 2BE.

Rowing

Crew racing as it is practised by rowing clubs and universities is a highly specialised sport demanding a high degree of physical fitness. Unless one is fortunate enough to live close to a river or lake it is unlikely that facilities and clubs open to rank beginners are easy to find. However, many will probably have the chance to take out the occasional skiff or rowing dinghy whilst on holiday, or if they live near water. Rowing is an excellent exercise as it combines the beauty of the surrounding area with aerobic benefit; it is therefore less monotonous than many other activities. It is sometimes possible to have coaching from experts, if one is able to find the right facilities. In this case it should be possible to graduate to competitive rowing with a club or college.

There are few activities that provide such all round exercise as rowing. Apart from its aerobic value, it is excellent for the leg muscles, shoulders, arms and back muscles.

For further details contact:

Amateur Rowing Association,
6 Lower Mall,
London, W6 9DJ.

Squash

This is now one of the most popular pastimes in Britain, being played by millions of both sexes. Its popularity is no doubt due in part to it being an indoor sport that can be played throughout the year. As a game it is relatively easy to learn, and the equipment not over-costly. It provides excellent exercise, demanding agility, co-ordination, power and stamina. Its value in respect of aerobic benefit is limited, due to the constant stoppages, however, if played for a long enough period at one time, benefit *will* accrue.

It bears repeating that one should get fit to play squash not play squash to get fit. The explosive nature of some actions in squash put a heavy demand on the heart and lungs for short bursts, and unless one is reasonably fit, should be played only at a reduced level. Unfortunately membership subscriptions of some clubs and court fees make it a rather expensive sport if played regularly.

A word of caution: due to the nature of the movements required, the game is not recommended for persons predisposed to backache.

For further information contact your local club or contact:

The Squash Rackets Association,
Francis House,
Francis Street,
London, SW1P 1DE.

or

Women's Squash Rackets Association,
345 Upper Richmond Road West,
Sheen,
London, SW14 8QN.

Swimming

This is one of the activities that most individuals, once they have become efficient, can continue for the rest of their lives. It is an exercise that does not require a great deal of power and yet provides aerobic benefit. As a competitive sport it is, unfortunately, generally limited to the younger age groups. However, some leisure centres and swimming clubs run events for veterans and special sessions for family groups. Even if one does not aspire to competitive swimming, great benefit can be derived from regular visits to the local pool, river or coast. Of course, during the winter season outdoor swimming is not recommended for those wishing to gain aerobic benefit. As a complementary activity to your regular workout, swimming will offer a suitable alternative to jogging or cycling if carried out regularly and practised for a sustained period.

The best stroke to use for sustained swimming is probably that which one finds easiest. It is recommended that swimming, if used as an exercise in fitness maintenance, should be carried out steadily for twenty to forty-five minutes without a rest. It does not require speed, but a steady continuous stroke. Even if one is not an expert, it is only a matter of regular practice to reach the required levels.

Further details are obtainable from:

Amateur Swimming Association,
Harold Fern House,
Derby Square,
Loughborough,
Leicestershire.

Orienteering

This is a fast growing sport which in many respects could be described as interval training with brains. It is well suited to the business executive who has attained a reasonably high level of physical fitness and wants to progress to a sporting challenge. The general aim is for participants to negotiate a course, usually in forest areas, defined by a number of control posts. Navigating by map and compass they attempt to do this by the best possible route and as quickly as possible. Courses usually range from two to eleven kilometres in length (straight line distance) with between six and twenty-five control points. The various features of the terrain shown on the map include the runnability, and this calls for constant pre-direction planning during the event.

This sport does not only attract athletes but is also geared for family groups, including children. The really fast runners very often get lost more easily, so giving a reasonable chance of victory to slower participants. Equipment required apart from the usual strip is a tracksuit, as full leg cover is compulsory, compass with protractor base, a whistle, map case, biro and your control card.

For futher information contact:

British Orienteering Federation,
41 Dale Road,
Matlock,
Derbyshire, DE4 3LT.

Judo

Strange as it may seem, this is not recognised as one of the martial arts. It is not so much a warlike practice, as a skill in off-balancing an opponent. Its principles are basically of a sporting nature with peaceful motives, although it can be an effective method of self-defence. Unlike wrestling it does not require great strength, but demands a very high degree of agility and timing. The training is strict and requires a lot of regular practice, leading to the attainment of coloured belts to denote one's level of proficiency. Higher grades or 'Dans' as they are called are the masters who have reached the level at which they are capable of highly sophisticated manoeuvres that require great skill in their execution.

There are many judo clubs situated all over Britain and these offer four categories of membership.

1. Club – single unit organisations.
2. Honorary Life – awarded as special recognition of service.
3. Individual – those that want to compete at Area, National or International level.
4. Junior – these should also be individual members if wishing to compete.

For further details contact:

The British Judo Association,
70 Brompton Road,
London, SW3 1DR.

or get in touch with your local sports or leisure centre.

5. The Martial Arts

Martial Arts is a term that strictly means ‘warlike practices’ and it has been used to cover such activities as quarterstaff, fencing and all forms of unarmed combat. Today the term is confined to the oriental forms of self defence such as aikido, jiu jitsu, karate, kung fu, kuk sool, tan soo do, tae kwon do, plus the Thai forms. These are hapkido, kendo, iaido, shorinji, kenijo, and wu shu. It should be remembered that all martial arts are methods of injuring or killing. Today in Britain they are practised as a form of sport or means of self defence. All forms of combat practices are potentially dangerous and should be strictly controlled in their usage, and taught only by experts. As a form of sport the movements can be extremely graceful requiring a high degree of balance and timing. Weapons are mostly confined to staves and where these are used protective clothing and face helmets are essential.

As a method of exercising their aerobic value is limited, but flexibility, agility and in some instances strength is enhanced. It is not always easy to find experienced coaches in some forms of martial art, but most large towns have a centre for the more popular methods.

For futher information contact:

The Martial Arts Commission,
Broadway House,
15/16 Deptford Broadway,
London, SE8 4PA.

IX

Relief of Boredom

The question of boredom frequently crops up throughout training programmes. Despite the fact that one can examine the points for and against the boredom factor, it does constitute one of the reasons for dropping out of the programme.

We offer some suggestions to minimise the drop-out rate resulting from boredom. They may add incentive to greater achievement within the programme.

Individual assistance

The individual should consciously attempt to try different ways of relieving boredom.

At home, for example, if you exercise with a static cycle, do you think of exercising in front of the television? Or do you consider looking out of the window when cycling, at some interesting activity going on around you, instead of a blank wall?

During the summer months you can move your cycle into the garden. Perhaps running on the spot is also assisted by a little thought with regard to surroundings and location. Some people like exercising in front of a mirror, others don't. Variety and change does a great deal to relieve the daily schedule.

External factors

There are a great many external factors that may influence the participant, that tend to relieve boredom. These are mainly associated with a group of people who are taking the programme together.

1. A regular re-test programme is essential.
2. Periodic competitions for charity.
   - Sponsor a FATTY! (a weight reduction competition)
   - Superstars
   - Fun runs
   - Marathons (full or half)
   - Reward for achievement (so many miles, weight achievement)
3. Publicity of achievement of personal goals.
4. Television and video programmes to relieve the monotony.

As you can see from the above there are many and varied ways to relieve the boredom factor. The difficulty is that no one can really identify why they get bored or what should be done about it.

All we can say for certain is that periodic changes or challenges seem to keep the interest alive in participants. The drop-out rate in the sponsored programme we refer to is relatively small.

The cup for a winner, the bottle of champagne to be shared with those who tried but did not win seem to give impetus to all concerned.

The re-test programme

The re-test programme when it appears on the horizon really does make the executive take a more active and dedicated approach towards his overall fitness and health.

A gentle reminder about a month or so in advance

ensures that he tries harder to raise the level of activity. The boredom factor seems to fall away for four to six weeks when the individual wants to see some improvement on his previous personal best performances. In addition, he may want to beat some colleagues' achievements who, in the recent past, have bettered their personal best – all good, clean competitive fun. It is not proposed to go into the specific details of the re-test programme at this stage, only to indicate that for some time prior to the re-test there are changes in the attitude and motivation of the participant.

Charity sponsorship

Donations to charity for best performance within age groups either by individuals or teams is an excellent way of alleviating boredom. Naturally, the first flush of enthusiasm is in-house, against one's close associates and colleagues. A further dimension is getting together to perform against others, whoever they may be. A gentle note of caution here, there must always be a sympathetic regard for the individual who does not wish to compete with others.

Personal recognition

Recognition for achievement whether it be personal or collective is an essential ingredient to overcoming the boredom factor. In this particular programme there is a good story to tell; it is a public relations officers' dream.

Television and Radio

A major step forward for early morning fitness people has been breakfast television, you can work-out and keep up-to-date with what is going on in the world. Very quickly you will also find that you can gear your work-out schedule to the programme. Not everyone's cup of tea, but there are a great many who are enthused by this added dimension.

Video, on the other hand is a matter of personal choice. Charged with enthusiasm for decathlon achievements, great marathons and a wide range of sporting activities, participants in the programme marvel at the achievements of the greats and are helped mentally to greater and better things.

In summary, there are many technical and innovative ways whereby the general fitness programme can be enhanced to relieve boredom and make participation so much more worthwhile.

X

Microcomputer Applications

There are three basic objectives to be kept in mind when putting the fitness programme on a microcomputer.

First, eliminating paperwork in the fitness environment.

Second, individual participation in answering the questionnaire, designing a programme with assistance, comparing your own performance over time, against your colleagues and against national averages.

Third, for the fitness supervisor to call up data with regard to re-test, individual or collective performance, regular reports, graphical and trend data on the total population.

The nature of the fitness programme is ideally suited to this kind of application.

The programme is simple and will enable the individual to be quickly educated and trained in all aspects of the fitness programme, at his or her own speed. They can go back to the terminal at leisure and continue the learning process. This approach keeps the programme interesting and gives increasing incentive to the participants.

The programme will be designed to cater for local needs but some of the basic requirements are:

1. Storage of individual questionnaire data.
2. Formatting a programme for each individual from a pre-determined range of possible protocols and exercises (pre-stretch, aerobics, power, post-stretch).

3. Comparison with prior work-outs – the individual can adjust the daily work-out according to his historical track. He only needs to input the present data, not repeat everything.
4. Having entered the basic data for the daily work-out, you can compare this data with the expected rate for the heart for the work-out, against a target. Other useful information can be quickly assessed; calories used-up, miles run or cycled, pace to be undertaken, how this individual work-out compares with the average (of the gymnasium or national).

Plenty of other data can also be entered, such as cholesterol count, EKG, date of last and next health screening, results of the last test, the date of the next test. Naturally, some individuals like to record more than others.

The kind of data that can be usefully recorded and compared is as follows:

	National Averages		*Authors' Programme*	
	Male	*Female*	*Male*	*Female*
Resting pulse rate	74	79	65	70
Blood pressure	130/82	131/82	122/76	118/69
Skinfold	15.5%	22.5%	15.8%	22.6%

TABLE 29

The design of the system has been developed in two parts taking into account the following requirements.

First, all the information relative to the daily work-outs of participants.

Second, the data base of all information to be stored relative to participants, comparative data, suggested diets, personalised recommendations.

The above system can easily be accommodated on most microcomputers. In addition, a useful capability is graphics software to display historical information, future aspirations and targets and a display of the ideal factors for each individual.

Appendix 1

Fitness, Facts And Fallacies

There are many common misunderstandings and myths in connection with physical exercise. Unfortunately, some of them can be attributed to doctors, sports coaches, amateur physical training instructors and other so-called experts. In this section we will pinpoint some of the facts and the more commonly held beliefs and put the records straight, using a question and answer format.

Q. Is it best to exercise first thing upon wakening?

A. No, just as a car engine needs to start slowly, so does the human body. It is probably better to exercise in the evening, or instead of lunch.

Q. If I stop exercising will I become fat?

A. Only if you were fat before and revert to your old habits, otherwise you will simply lose muscle tone.

Q. I am a female – if I use weights will I develop big muscles?

A. It is unlikely unless the weights you use are very heavy, allowing less than six repetitions. Small weights will help tone up your muscles and enhance your natural curves.

Q. I can touch my toes without bending my knees, is this a good sign of fitness?

A. No, many very fit persons cannot do this, just as many unfit persons *can* do it. In any case it is a dangerous movement and should never be included in tests of fitness.

Q. If I run at 10 m.p.h. for 6 minutes will this give me the same aerobic benefit as running at 6 m.p.h. for 10 minutes?

A. No, although your pulse rate will be elevated at 10 m.p.h. it will not be sustained for long enough to provide much aerobic benefit. A longer period of endurance even if at lower speeds is generally more beneficial aerobically.

Q. Unless exercises hurt they are not doing much good, is this right?

A. No, a thousand times no. If one exercises to the point of actual pain, it is probably doing far more harm than good. Exercises should be carried out gently and rythmically.

Q. If I work-out with weights will I become muscle-bound?

A. Only if it is the only exercise that you do. The expression merely implies that the bulk of muscle tissue impinges upon joint flexibility and co-ordination is affected.

Q. I want to lose weight, if I do weight training will it do the trick?

A. Unless you also diet, it is more likely that you will gain weight, as muscles weigh more than fat.

Q. If I exercise regularly, will it prevent me from having a heart attack?

A. No. If your general history predisposes you to possible heart attack, exercises will not prevent it, but it may well help you to recover from it and lessen the effects.

Q. I sweat profusely when I undertake exercise, is this a bad sign?

A. No, on the contrary, it shows that your temperature regulating centre is working efficiently.

Q. I sometimes feel palpitations in my chest, is this a sign of heart disease?

A. Not necessarily, palpitations are quite common in quite fit people and may be caused by stress, cigarette smoking, over-indulgence, coffee drinking and many other non-sinister reasons. However, it is perhaps wise to speak to your doctor.

Q. Should I use a specific breathing pattern when I exercise and run?

A. It is not necessary to concern yourself too much with breathing techniques, however breath holding for long periods during explosive activity is not recommended.

Q. When I run I sometimes experience pain in my side – should I stop running?

A. This is probably due to diaphragm spasm causing 'stitch'. Unless it is very painful, it may only be necessary to slow down. Sometimes it helps to press over the painful region for a minute or so. A change of breathing pattern may also help.

Q. Fat people are better swimmers than lean persons, is this true?

A. In long distance events over three miles, it is usually fatter individuals that do best, this is because heat retention is better. Because fat floats better than muscle there is less resistance. However, in shorter explosive events, leaner persons usually do best.

Q. I am a diabetic, are there any limitations to the level at which I exercise?

A. You must consult your physician, but if your diabetes is under control there is very little reason why you should not exercise within normal limits.

Q. Should I stop my exercise programme during menstruation?

A. You must be guided by how you feel, but normally there should be no reason to stop, although it may be wise to slow it down.

Q. My exercise pulse-rate ceiling has been set at 160 beats per minute, is it dangerous for me to exceed this?

A. Until you have reached a fairly high level of fitness, it would be wise to keep within this limit. After that your exercise tolerance will be such that you will find it difficult to even reach your ceiling.

Q. Should I ignore feelings of gross fatigue or unusual aches and pains when I exercise?

A. **Absolutely not.** In all cases of doubt with regard to your personal well-being you *must* seek medical advice.

Q. I am over 50 years of age and have not exercised for several years, is it too late for me to start?

A. Absolutely not, but remember to have a medical check first, start slowly, and do not try to compete. Eventually, you should be fit enough to run several miles and to start enjoying life again.

Q. My doctor has told me that I have osteo-arthritis in my hips, I think exercise may help, am I right?

A. Yes! Gentle mobilising exercises during times when the hips are not too painful will help prevent deterioration. However, more energetic exercise should not be attempted without your doctor's advice.

Appendix 2

Dietary Considerations

It is not in the scope of this book to offer specialised diets; there are already countless books on this subject and much has been written about the subject of slimming. It is perhaps helpful, however, to discuss the wider implications of food intake with regard to exercise.

It is very often difficult for the executive to get out of the so-called 'business lunch', but waiters in restaurants and hotels do not force their clients to eat huge amounts of the wrong foods. Most places have a wide variety of salads and fish dishes that, when prepared raw or boiled, are less harmful than grilled and fried foods. It is quite clear that for the human body to survive, calorie intake must be at least sufficient to cope with energy expenditure. But it is equally clear that in an affluent society most exceed their calorie requirements, in other words most eat too much or exercise too little.

Obesity is said to be that state in which men have more than 20% body-fat and women more than 26%. It is perhaps surprising that many people exceed these figures even though their calorie intake is not excessive. This is often due to a slow metabolic rate combined with a very low physical activity. The answer is more activity rather than lowering the calorie intake. Some argue that although they have very active life-styles and take part in regular sporting or exercise programmes, they are still overweight. Firstly, this may be due to good musculature (muscles weigh heavier than fat). Secondly, it may be that their calorie intake is still above their needs. The answer for the latter is simply a matter of eating less even though their level of physical activity increases their appetite. It is a fact that *intense* levels of muscular exercise will in fact decrease appetite by inhibiting the supply of blood to the digestive system. This should not be considered abnormal, and often it is an excellent method of suppressing the desire to eat. In other words, if you are eating in excess of your calorie requirements, when you feel hungry, exercise at high levels, instead of eating more.

For many who live an executive life-style, eating is an important social occasion when entertaining friends, business acquaintances and prospective clients, and there is no reason why this should not be so. The important consideration is in choosing the right menu, which will suit the occasion and yet not add to the problems of dietary control. In this circumstance there are several ways by which success can be achieved, but first a few guidelines should be observed:

1. Boil rather than fry or grill
2. Cut away all the fat
3. Eat fish rather than meat
4. Use vegetables raw if possible
5. Use fresh fruit rather than tinned
6. Eat desserts that do not require sugar
7. Do not add oil to salads
8. Drink dry rather than sweet
9. White meat has less calories than red meat

There are many recipes for meals that are colourful, tasty and satisfying and yet low in calories. In particular, consider some of the Asiatic dishes based on boiled rice and fish, or even vegetarian-type meals using raw vegetables and natural foods. Whatever the menu, weight control is essentially a matter of balance, not only between energy intake and expenditure, but also in food values.

It is important to remember that the three main foods are: fats, proteins and carbohydrates, and most of the things we eat contain at least one of these, plus small amounts of the vital minerals and vitamins that we need. A constant diet that lacks any one of these constituents will inevitably lead to one of the deficiency illnesses. Here are a few examples of foods that yield high quantities of fats, proteins or carbohydrates.

Fats: which are the highest in calories, providing energy:

Oil or lard
Butter
Bacon
Cheddar Cheese
Vegetable Fats such as Margarine and Olive Oil

Proteins: important in tissue growth:

Green Vegetables
Eggs
Milk
Cheese
Lean Meat
Oatmeal
Chicken
Fish

Carbohydrates: very important for energy in the form of glucose, which is the result of its breakdown in the digestive system:

Cereals
Dates
Prunes
Macaroni
Sugar
Most Vegetables

Most of the necessary vitamins and minerals are found in large enough quantities in our food to satisfy our needs. There is little evidence to suggest that we need to take extra vitamins in pills, or that, if we do, they will benefit us.

Carbohydrate Loading

As has been stated on page 186, carbohydrates are broken down to form glycogen which provides energy to the working muscles. In long distance athletic events such as the Marathon and other sports requiring a high degree of stamina, the glycogen is reduced to very low proportions causing exhaustion.

There is much evidence today to support the idea of carbohydrate loading. This is done by the ingestion of only proteins and fats for several days during training. This reduces glycogen drastically. Then three to four days before the event a diet very high in carbohydrates is taken so that a huge amount of carbohydrates is stored in the liver and muscles. This diet is not recommended for events lasting less than half an hour. Generally speaking, the basic needs for most persons following a sports or fitness training programme should consist of 45% – 50% carbohydrates, 30% – 40% fats and 15% – 20% proteins. Adequate intake of water is of course essential. On this diet there should be no need to take extra minerals or vitamins.

Appendix 3

Equipment Portfolio

Personal

Your Strip

This consists of your exercise apparel, shorts, singlet or running vest, supports and socks. In some specialised fitness activity it will consist of clothing adapted specifically for it.

This is largely a matter of personal choice, and one must select from experience, but for those individuals that are newly embarking upon a fitness or running programme, a few words of advice. Chafing is probably one of the worst problems of clothing, especially in activities that involve a particular pattern of movement over long periods, such as running or cycling. This can be caused by clothing that is too tight or too course and by seams and stitching that are frequently brought into contact with the skin. When selecting your shorts and vest make sure that they are easy fitting, that friction points are not heavily stitched by seams or by badges and embroidery. The materials are best if they are soft and sweat-absorbent, and woollen socks are generally superior and more comfortable than those of man-made fibres. Leotards, although suitable for general physical exercise and movement are not recommended for running.

Some sports manufacturers now have bras especially made for high level activity. It would seem however, that very few women athletes are subject to breast pain or nipple soreness through the wearing of ordinary bras. It is suggested that these should be made of absorbent material and constructed with seamless cups, shoulder straps that do not drift and clasps that will not cause irritation.

Some men prefer briefs rather than jock straps and that is a personal matter, but whatever is worn as a means of support, it is a wise precaution against chafing to apply Vaselene to the areas of the groin where friction may occur. Sweat-shirts and track-suits are seldom used during physical activity by most runners. However, during the winter months it would seem wise to have these ready for the coldest temperatures. Man-made fibres are less absorbent, less comfortable, and generally less warm than wool or cotton mixture. For cold insulation before and after competition or activity, track suits are invaluable. Sweat-shirts and track-suit tops should be fitted with a hood if one is subjected to very cold temperatures.

Your Running Shoe

This is the most important item of your personal equipment and therefore great care should be taken in your selection of footwear.

First, an analysis of your running action with regard to the foot is essential so that one may spot possible abnormalities in one's own style. The heel strike is generally best if it occurs centrally but it is not unusual to have a slight lateral tilt. As the weight of the body comes over the foot it is transmitted along the outer border onto the ball (or metatarsal heads) finally flattening out to push off from the big toe, as the weight passes ahead of the foot. A glance at the heels of your old shoes will indicate by the areas of wear whether or not your heel strike is right, and the soles will show the weight transferance pattern.

Excessive wear along the outer curve of the heel would indicate that there is too much inversion (turning the sole of the foot inwards). It is relatively rare to see wear occurring at the inner edge of the heel, but if this is so it indicates an eversion of the foot (turning the sole outwards). In both cases the torsion stresses which are imposed on the ankle ligaments and to the achilles tendon may result in injury.

It must be remembered that during running the heel strikes the surface with a force two or three times greater than the runner's body weight. This strike happens several thousand times to both feet every time a run of two miles or more is undertaken. The force is then transmitted into the ankle joint, up the shaft of the leg bone and into the knee joint. It is little wonder therefore, that runners frequently suffer bruised heels, shin soreness, sprained ankle and knee pain. Stress fractures often occur in the small bones of the foot and ligamentous strains are common along the sole of the foot.

Running shoes today have become very sophisticated with various designs of insole, wedges, heel counters and re-inforced uppers. What then should the buyer look for? This is a question that cannot be fully answered because it is only by experience of the individual that the right shoe can be found. The make and design that is right for one person may be entirely unsuited for another. However there are several points that can be made which will act as a guide in the selection of a shoe best suited to your style of running.

To help in the prevention of excessive inversion or eversion one should look for a shoe with a more rigid heel box. This should be of the correct width so that the heel fits snugly into it. Bruising and stress fractures occurring in the small bones of the foot are often the result of inadequate cushioning. This is extremely important in runners who take to the roads or habitually run on hard surfaces. One should look for a good thickness of sole and wedging, especially at the heel, (it is recommended that this be at least half an inch thick with shock absorbent qualities). Nowadays one can buy specially made inserts that are designed to absorb shock and have proved very effective in preventing injury. These are made of a substance that, because of its visco-elastic properties, closely resembles the texture of human muscle tissue. For persons who are predisposed towards back ache, complain of knee, ankle or foot pain when running, the inserts very often prove to be a sensible precaution. These visco-elastic inserts are made in various sizes and for different parts of the foot. Most of the larger sports stores, especially those that tend to specialise in running and athletics will be able to help, advise and supply.

Flexibility is also a very important factor in the design of a running shoe; although it is critical that heel boxes and some parts of the the uppers should offer firm support, shoes that are flexible across the forefoot are less likely to cause certain foot problems such as metatarsalgia and plantar fasciitis (see sports injuries and their treatment on page 199).

A good test of shoe flexibility is to try to bring the toe of the upper to the heel of the upper, if this is too easy, the shoes are generally not as robust as they ought to be. On the other hand, if the test requires an element of strain, it may be due to too much rigidity in the design. Remember that flexibility of a shoe tends to increase with wear and tear, so in performing the test, one should look for a degree or two of resistance.

Shoe fitting is vital for comfort, and most persons will have their own ideas about this, yet many cases of foot and toe problems can be attributed to wrong sizing. It should be remembered that most persons' feet tend to get larger with age, especially in the width. As a general rule the length should allow a clear inch between the tip of one's large toe and the end of the inside shoe.

The width should make a snug envelope for the foot without cramping the toes or compressing the instep. Laces can often cause problems by being too tightly tied or because the tongue of the shoe is too short and insufficiently padded.

Finally, a word about weight, a lot of enthusiastic joggers and runners are prepared to sacrifice quality for lightness. It is true that most good quality shoes are made to be as light as possible and that is good, but occasionally one finds a shoe that has been made almost weightless by the lack of sole thickness, and these will not dissipate shock. It is also recommended that one should look for a shoe in a higher rather than a lower price range.

Gynnasium Equipment

Designing and Planning the Executive Gymnasium

'In House' fitness is one of the fastest growing areas in today's fitness boom. It is important to realise though, that the commercial or corporate fitness gymnasium is a very different concept to the home gym: the design and planning criteria are more akin to the objectives of planning a factory layout or production line rather than a small R and D department.

The final layout and combination of all the necessary equipment has also been likened to the principles of selecting a computer. When the final choice is right the hardware remains essentially the same but the programmes change depending on your objectives. So let us examine the objectives of an executive gym:

1. *To Provide Total Fitness for All Users*
   A well balanced layout and the right type of equipment in the correct environment will enable programmes to be designed for improvements in: speed, strength, aerobic fitness and flexibility, i.e. improved job-related human performance.
2. *To Exercise the Maximum Number of Users in a Limited Space*
   Space, whether it be in a corporate organisation, hotel, or commercial health studio, costs money. Careful planning to obtain efficient use of that space by maximising throughput of personnel and balancing changing room space with cosmetic fitness space and exercise space is essential.
3. *To Provide Maximum Revenue (Commercial Gymnasia)*
   The whole future of a commercial venture will rest upon a reasonable return on capital. This return will not be forthcoming if it is not considered at the gymnasium planning stage.
4. *To Improve Users' Physical Appearance*
   Fitness (objective 1) is quite different from physical appearance, a loss or gain of weight or vastly improved physical shape is possible, within a relatively short period of time.
5. *Rehabilitate After Illness or Injury*
   The best method, one which we hope you will be following, is prevention rather than cure. However, strokes, heart attacks, and industrial and sporting injuries do occur, with the corresponding loss of millions of working hours per year.

Specialist equipment can be designed into the gymnasium to cater for individual rehabilitation programmes, however, only suitably qualified instructors liaising with medical personnel must supervise the programmes.

The variations in the type of design and programmes are immense and are governed by the type of organisation, division or tasks fitting known job descriptions. For instance a coal face worker employed by the N.C.B. has a different requirement from an N.C.B. office-bound executive. Yet the coal face worker may have broadly similar requirements to a seemingly unrelated job – a fireman. And by the same token a chief fire officer's task has become largely sedentary, and would therefore be broadly aligned with the N.C.B. executive.

So it is possible to categorise broadly and produce a middle of the road design, resulting in a gymnasium suitable for most types. Fine tuning is given by individualising the programme. Here are three condensed case studies to illustrate the point clearly:

Mid-Glamorgan Fire Department

During 1983 a unique experiment was set up between Mid-Glamorgan Fire Service and Powersport International Limited. The experiment started with an on-site analysis of the physical tasks carried out by firemen, categorising them under the headings; Aerobic Fitness, Dynamic Strength, Speed, Static Strength and Explosive Strength. It was found that firemen were placed under severe physical loads, lifting in excess of 300 lbs., sprinting, wearing full equipment, climbing ladders, etc. from a cold body situation. Results were tabulated and further analysed to show muscle function, and then exercises were allocated to improve the function.

Only at the termination of this stage did a final design for equipment materialise.

The experiment began: Four watches of firemen engaged in a four day a week split programme of 'In House' fitness training on a Multigym System. Results were measured against a practical test battery aligned to the priority requirements of firemen (1. Dynamic Strength, 2. Aerobic Fitness, 3. Speed).

1. Bench Press – 10 repetitions maximum.
2. Squat (90°Leg Bend) – 10 repetitions maximum.
3. Number of sit-ups in one minute.
4. Vertical Jump.
5. Shuttle Run.

Body Measurement – weight only in kgs.

Physical results were highly satisfactory with all individuals making measurable progress between 5%-35%, as measured on the test battery.

More remarkable, however, were spin-off results analysed by Brigade Training Officer Eric Clark:

1. Reduced Absenteeism.
2. Improved Morale.
3. Improved Performance.
4. Fewer Accidents.

Rank Xerox Scheme

During the early 1970s Gerry Rickards approached Peter Lay, designer and founder of the Multigym System to plan mutually the first corporate executive gymnasium for Rank Xerox's Euston Road Headquarters. During the ensuing decade the gymnasium has become a model visited by hundreds of corporation fitness disciples and a legend in the 'In House' fitness field. Rank Xerox have also improved upon the initial plan with each of their gymnasia, since there is little doubt the original was essentially right. Rickards and Lay planned an all-round gymnasium catering for aerobic fitness, strength and speed, using a 12 station Multigym and wall unit configuration, treadmills, static cycles, and a jogging programme. Other aspects such as rehabilitation in all forms were Rickards' speciality and he quotes remarkable results.

Testimony to the huge success of the 'first' of its kind in the U.K. corporate world was the fact that the Xerox board voted for further gymnasia to be built in the group. A decision hard-headed successful businessmen did not take lightly.

North Sea Oil Rigs

Most of the companies operating oil rigs in the North Sea have installed Multigyms for the use of their personnel. Here the purpose of installing the equipment is twofold, (a) the nature of the job requires that operatives be extremely fit and (b) with such a captive audience in so small a space the Multigym is a valuable recreational aid.

Some facts which govern the scheme:

1. What space is available (Dimension)? Don't forget room height.
2. How much capital is available?
3. Can it be increased?
4. Can I use off balance sheet finance (Leasing)?
5. What income is forecast? (for commercial organisations).
6. How many users per hour at peak times?
7. Men or women users, or both?
8. How many instructors will I need?
9. Can I provide maintenance or do I need agreement with the supply company?
10. Will the floor stand the load?
11. Am I prepared to assemble or fix equipment to walls?
12. Is there a weight-bearing wall suitable for fixing?

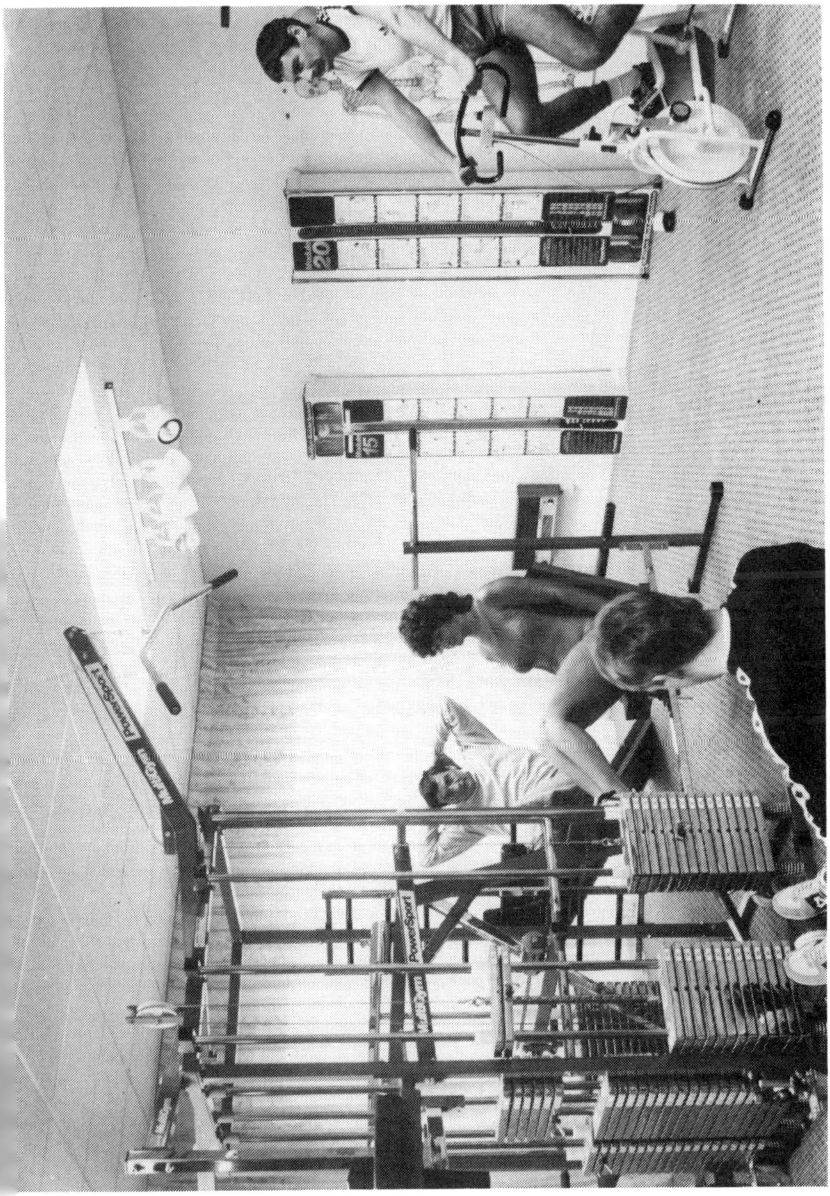

Appendix 4

Sports Injuries And Treatment

In any form of sport or physical exercise there exists the risk of injury, indeed there are some who feel that this is the very risk that gives the spice to the activity. This thought is vividly expressed in the following lines by Adam Lindsay Gordon.

No game was ever yet worth a rap
For a rational man to play.
Into which no accident, no mishap
Could possibly find its way.

However, by diligent observance of safety rules in exercise regime, injuries are much less likely to occur. It is not always possible of course, to predict the unexpected that may result in accidents.

The obvious and sensible course of action following injury is to report to a doctor, but it may be several hours before a medical examination actually takes place. The first few hours following injury sustained in sport or exercise are very often the most crucial in terms of speedy recovery. Here is a brief list of ways in which you may be able to act immediately an injury occurs. It must be stressed that this advice is intended only to apply up to 36 hours following injury, thereafter medical opinion must be sought.

1. *Soft tissue bruising*
   This can sometimes be quite severe and should thus be treated seriously. Apply cold water or ice wrapped in a towel. This should be done without delay and continued for approximately 15 minutes, after which the part should be kept as immobile

as possible. Apply warmth at intervals after the first 2 or 3 hours.
DO NOT MASSAGE DIRECTLY OVER THE SITE OF THE INJURY.

2. *Bone and joint bruising*
Treatment as above, but in the case of joints, swelling is more likely to be a complication, immobilisation should be re-inforced by the application of a bandage extending well above and below the joint. If the injury involves a limb, then this should be elevated so that the effects of gravity on excess fluid are to some extent nullified. In this type of bruising, pain may continue long after signs of the bruising have disappeared.

3. *Swollen and painful upper limb* (Where fracture is not suspected)
Apply ice for the first ten or fifteen minutes, then rest the arm in a sling applied so that the hand is higher than the elbow.

4. *Swollen and painful lower limb* (Where fracture is not suspected)
Treatment as for upper limb. Rest with the leg elevated so that the heel is higher than the hip and the back of the knee supported.

5. *Suspected Fractures* (Where skin is unbroken)
Immediate immobilisation by strapping arm to body, or leg to leg if this is possible without increasing injury. Keep warm, await arrival of doctor.

6. *Open Fractures* (Where skin is broken)
Stem flow of blood by application of a dressing, and if possible, without worsening injury, elevate the part. Then treat as above.
LOSE NO TIME IN SENDING FOR A DOCTOR.

7. *Metatarsalgia*
   In this, pain is felt under the ball of the foot, sometimes caused by stress fracture or bruising of the bony underlying parts. Treatment. Rest from running until condition settles down. Consider different shoes.

8. *Plantar fasciitis*
   This is a painful condition affecting the sole of the foot especially close to the heel. It is generally due to an inflammation of the fascial layers under the skin. This is often caused by over-use such as in Marathon training and by ill-suited running shoes. Treatment. Rest from running until the condition settles down and also consider changing your running shoes. Sometimes heel-pads are helpful when worn inside the shoe.

9. *Tendon Strains*
   These strains can be recognised by localised soreness or aching along the course of the tendon during its use. This is caused by over-use of muscles particularly in unaccustomed activity. Running or jumping on the toes is a common cause of Achilles Tendon strain. Treatment is immediate rest from the activity responsible.

10. *Cramp*
    Localised cramp occurring in a muscle is best relieved by sustained stretching of the spasm by extension or flexion of the joints upon which the muscle acts. Severe cramp affecting several muscle groups may be due to excessive salt loss in sweating, especially in hot climates. The administration of a tumbler full of salt water should not be delayed.

11. *Heat Stroke*
    In this the temperature of the body rises to a very high level and there is a feeling of nausea and dizziness. There may be muscular twitchings and shivering. Immediate efforts must be made to reduce the body temperature. This may be done by immersion in cold water with the body wrapped in a towel or blanket. Ice packs, if available, should be applied.

12. *Muscle and Ligament tears*
    Recognised by a sudden severe pain on movement of the part involved. Immediate rest and immobilisation of the part should follow early application of ice or water. Immobilisation is best achieved by the application of a pressure bandage extending well above and below the site of injury. A pressure bandage of two or three crepe or similar bandages between each of which is a thick layer of cotton wool is wrapped around the limb. Each bandage is applied with increasing tension but still enabling normal blood circulation to take place. Elevation of the injured part will aid recovery.
    DO NOT BEAR WEIGHT ON AN INJURED LIMB.

13. *Fainting*
    Loosen tight clothing, keep head low and raise the legs. Do not administer fluids until full recovery has taken place.
    DO NOT PUMP HEAD BETWEEN LEGS.

14. *Chest pains while exercising*
    Discontinue exercise immediately, lie down, keep warm and await arrival of doctor.

GENERAL RULES TO BE APPLIED IN FIRST AID

- Send for medical aid as soon as possible if indicated.
- Treat the most urgent condition first. In order, these are:
  (a) cessation of breathing
  (b) profuse bleeding
  (c) shock
- Never apply ice directly onto skin.
- Do not give anything by mouth to an unconscious person.

Appendix 5

Questionnaires

FITNESS QUESTIONNAIRE

1. *Personal*

NAME: AGE: HEIGHT:

PRESENT WEIGHT: TITLE:

LOCATION:

2. *Health Factors*

	YES	NO
• Have you ever had a serious injury, illness or operation?		
• Do you have, or have you ever been treated for.		
– Shortness of breath?		
– High blood pressure?		
– Pains in the chest?		
– Dizziness or fainting?		
– Diabetes?		

3. *Job and non job related activities*

	High	*Medium*	*Low*
• How would you rate the amount of physical activity:–			
– at work?			
– during leisure time?			
• How would you rate your present overall physical level?			
• What percentage of time do you travel?			

	YES	NO
• Do you smoke?		

TABLE 30

PROGRAMME QUESTIONNAIRE

Comments

1. *Do you participate in any sporting activity?*
   - competitively
   - recreation
   - keep fit only

2. *When did you last participate actively in sport?*
   - 1 year ago
   - 2 years ago
   - over 5 years

3. *What sports did you participate in?*
   - aerobic
   - power
   - flexibility

4. *What activities do you most enjoy?*
   - running
   - cycling
   - weight training
   - other

5. *What do you want to gain from the programme?*
   - weight loss
   - aerobic endurance
   - increased muscular power
   - flexibility
   - all round health and well-being

TABLE 31

Appendix 6

Training Log

DAILY ROUTINE (Individual)

- *PRE-STRETCH (5 minutes)*

- *CIRCLE*
  - Head
  - Shoulder

- *TWIST*
  - Side
  -

- *STRETCH*
  - Side
  - Thigh
  - Hamstring/Calf
  - Ankle

- *AEROBIC (Cardio-Vascular Progress)*

DATE:

METHOD:

SPEED:

ENDURANCE:

TABLE 32

POWER (Multigym)

Date of Exercise ....

Station	*Number Of Repetitions and Weight*	*Repetitions*	*Weight*	*Repetitions*	*Weight*
A	Leg Press				
B	Pull Down				
C	Bicep Curl				
D	Shoulder Press				
E	Chinning				
F	Bench Press				
G	Inclined Sit-Ups				
H	Dips				
I	Wrist Roll				
J	Hyper-Extension				
K	Hamstring Pull				
L	Leg Extension				

- *POST-STRETCH (Free Activity)*

- Step-Ups
- Skipping
- Static Cycle
- Walking
- Table/Padder Tennis
- Punch Ball
- Rowing
- Medicine Ball
- Ski-ing

TABLE 33

TRAINING LOG
WEEKLY/MONTHLY PROGRESS CHART
(Individual and Supervised)

- *FITNESS LEVEL ASSESSMENT*

NAME: .... AGE: ....

SOMATOTYPE ....

WEEK:	*1*	*2*	*3*	*4*	*5*	*MONTH END*	*TARGET*
DATE:							
METHOD: Treadmill/Cycle or any other aerobic activity							
RESTING PULSE RATE:							
BLOOD PRESSURE:							
SKIN FOLD:							
PEAK FLOW:							
ACTIVITY: Time on treadmill or cycle at miles per hour							
PULSE RATE – AFTER EXERCISE – RECOVERY							
WEIGHT:							

TABLE 34

TRAINING LOG – WEEKLY GRAPHICAL

Method: Treadmill/Cycle

Recovery Rate

Date ....

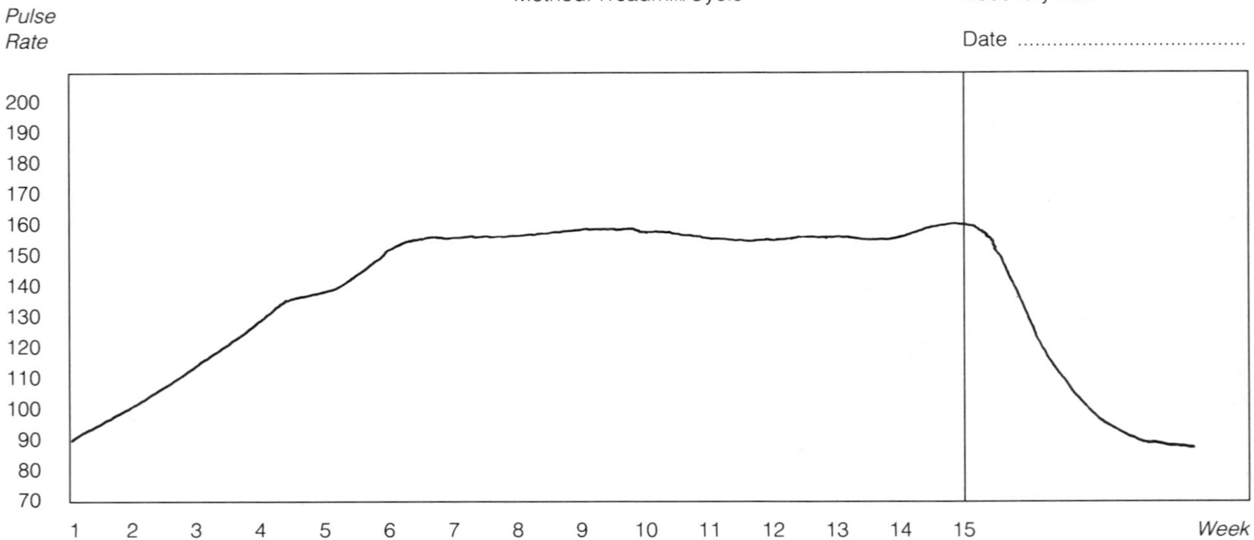

TABLE 35

CUMULATIVE MILES

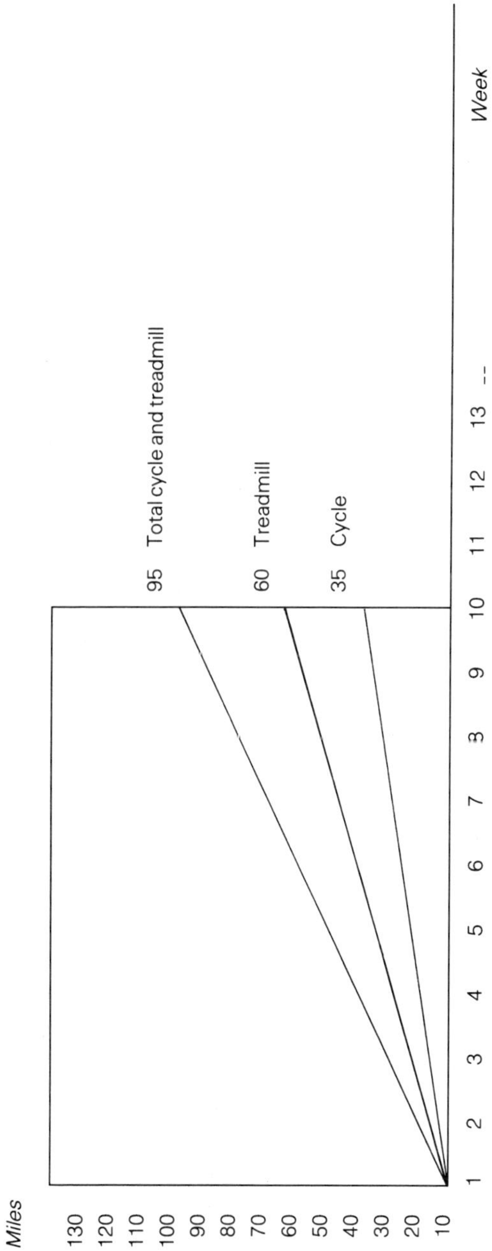

TABLE 36

Appendix 7

Preventive Medicine – A Practical Reality

That prevention is better than cure is one of the oldest and most readily accepted adages.

Sadly, when it comes to applying this philosophy to health maintenance, one soon sees that practical medicine is heavily weighted towards cure and that most people, including some doctors, are unconcerned with health risks and indifferent to minimising them until something goes wrong. Of course there are exceptions; mass radiography of the chest, cervical cytology and immunisation against crippling diseases in infancy.

The concept of regularly examining well people with the aim of keeping them well is relatively new. The Americans call it Automated Multiphasic Health Testing (AMHT), 'automated' because most systems for applying large numbers of tests to large numbers of people rely on computers for the recording, collating and quality controlling of test data.

In the U.K. this type of medicine has been functioning for about 20 years and was pioneered by Dr. H. Beric Wright at the Institute of Directors in London. The unit he established merged with BUPA in January 1972 and has developed in both expertise and popularity (over 250,000 patients have been seen by BUPA Medical Centres). Patients are examined in relation to their whole environment, social, domestic, work, as well as their purely physical and psychological state, because this type of medicine aims not only to prolong life but also to improve its quality.

The logistics and economics of preventive medicine merit close scrutiny. If the philosophy were to be applied to the whole population two things would have to happen: first, a major educational campaign to train people to think in terms of basic health maintenance *while they are still well* would be required; second, the health service would have to reorientate itself to the task of applying preventive measures rather than curative. No system is perfect and we could never attain a situation where illness and disease ceased to exist, but there are many common conditions, e.g. respiratory disease, proneness to coronary heart attack, breast cancer, which can be detected and forestalled or, at least, reduced in severity of effect. Such measures would relieve the over-burdened state system of both costs and manpower commitment by reducing the numbers of in-patients and the length of stay in hospital for those who did have to have treatment. This ideal is a long way from being realised by the Department of Health acknowledged the possibilities in a report published as early as 1976. *(Prevention & health everybody's business*. HMSO 1976).

The principles of screening populations for covert or pre-symptomatic disease are as follows:

1. The condition sought should be an important health problem.
2. There should be an accepted treatment for patients with recognised disease.
3. Facilities for diagnosis and treatment should be available.
4. There should be a recognisable latent or early symptomatic stage.
5. There should be a suitable test or examination.
6. The test should be acceptable to the population.
7. The natural history of the condition, including development from latent to declared disease, should be adequately understood.
8. There should be an agreed policy on whom to treat as patients.

9. The cost of case-finding (including diagnosis and treatment of patients diagnosed) should be economically balanced in relation to possible expenditure on medical care as a whole.
10. Case-finding should be a continuing process and not a 'once and for all project'.

It is difficult if not impossible to meet all these criteria but two diseases stand out above all others as prime candidates for a health screening programme in the so-called civilised Western democracies. These are Coronary Heart Disease (CHD) and Breast Cancer.

In the U.K. CHD is the biggest killer of middle-aged men. One in 10 of 35 year old males will not live to collect their pension because of coronary heart disease and 1 in 4 will suffer from it before age 65.

Coronary-prone individuals can be identified on a risk factor basis which takes up to eight factors into account These are family history, electro-cardiograph of heart function, blood pressure, weight, exercise (or, usually, lack of it!), blood fat level (cholesterol), smoking, stress. Some of these are unmodifiable, notably family history, but others can be corrected by good advice well followed or by drug therapy or a combination of both. Certainly the person who regulates life style to avoid the major hazards can significantly reduce the chance of developing coronary heart disease in middle years.

Among women, the equivalent to heart disease in men is breast cancer which affects 1 in 17 women in the U.K. at some time during their lives. Over 13,000 women die each year in the U.K. from breast cancer compared with approximately 2,500 from cervical cancer. Between the ages of 35 and 54 breast cancer kills more women in the U.K. than any other single disease. After that age heart disease takes over as the major cause of death in women as in men. In younger women gynaecological examination reveals more problems than breast examination and most of these can again be dealt with quite simply, frequently by good advice.

All these diseases are eminently treatable if caught in their early stages, Electrocardiograph, blood pressure recording, blood lipid profile and weight measurements help to identify the coronary prone individual, while soft x-ray mammography, manual palpation and training in self-examination are effective in early detection of breast abnormalities. Quite apart from these killer diseases many respiratory and musculo-skeletal disorders are brought to light by health screening which, additionally, may include tests of hearing, vision, lung function, chest x-rays, urinalysis and pulse rate. All these tests go to produce a detailed profile of a person's existing state of health and likely risk of future disease.

BUPA's Medical Centres are typical of the health screening systems available in the U.K. having been established in 1970 and with experience going back six years before that.

Under the BUPA screening system results of all the tests are sent to the patient's own doctor who is responsible for follow-up and treatment where necessary. One third of all patients attending have some form of abnormality. Most of these are simple problems, perhaps overweight or heavy smoking, but one in five has conditions requiring something more than a bit of good advice, while 4% have serious abnormalities.

The moral is clear; prudent prevention where disease is concerned has to be more sensible than trying to cure conditions which might have been prevented, by applying to our minds and bodies even the basic amount of care and maintenance we give to our cars or other material possessions.

Much has now been written on the subject of preventive

medicine and authorities are still divided on the value of it. Probably in the U.K. 100,000 or more people each year pay to receive the undoubted reassurance that health screening can provide. This is a relatively small number but, if you talk to anyone who has undergone health screening, you will almost certainly find that they place great value on the help and reassurance it provides.

Useful reading

'Facts About' series published by BUPA Medical Centre Ltd.

BREASTS and the importance of breast examination
CANCER and getting it into perspective
CORONARY THROMBOSIS–avoid or live with it
DRINKING and how to control it
EXECUTIVE TRAVEL and how to survive
THE MENOPAUSE and how to live through it
OBESITY and how to control your weight
POSTURE & EXERCISE and how to keep moving
PRE-MENSTRUAL SYNDROME
SLEEP and REST
SMOKING and how to stop

These booklets, currently priced at 85p each, postage paid, contain many other useful references.

GLOSSARY

Aerobic Having molecular oxygen present.

Anaerobic Lacking molecular oxygen.

Cardiac Pertaining to the heart.

Cardio-vascular Pertaining to the heart and blood vessels.

Cardio-respiratory Pertaining to the heart and lungs.

Circulo-respiratory Pertaining to the blood vessels and lungs.

Chronic Persisting over a long period of time.

Coma position That in which an unconscious person is placed to avoid complications such as choking. It is also considered to be the most relaxing position.

Congenital Existing at, and usually before birth: referring to conditions that are present at birth regardless of their cause.

Connective tissue Body tissues that connect more actively functioning tissues such as cartilage, bone and muscle.

Cybernetics The science of the processes of communication and control in the person and in the machine.

Cyclical Pertaining to, or occurring in a cycle or cycles.

Diastolic Pertaining to the period of relaxation of the heart before the contraction.

Electro-cardiograph An instrument for measuring the electric currents generated by the heart.

Ergometer An apparatus, such as a static cycle, used to measure the muscular and respiratory effects of exercise.

Ergonomics The science relating to man and his work embodying the anatomic, physiologic, psychologic and mechanical principles affecting the efficient use of human energy.

Extensibility The maximum safe length to which a muscle may be stretched.

Excursion Movements occurring from a normal, or rest, position of a moveable part such as the chest wall in respiration.

Genetic Pertaining to birth or origin.

Hamstring The tendons of the muscles at the back of the thigh.

Heelcord The achilles tendon especially the lower part before it inserts into the heel bone.

Hyperventilation A state in which there is an increased amount of air entering the lungs, resulting in an oxygen saturation of the blood cells.

Hypoglycaemia An abnormally diminished content of glucose in the blood.

Isometric Contraction of muscles without joint movement.

Isotonic Contraction of muscles with joint movement caused by the muscle action.

Lactic acid One of the substances that accumulates from the breakdown of energy-producing chemicals during muscular exertion.

Lateral Pertaining to a side away from the mid-line of the body.

Lumbar Pertaining to the lower back.

Metabolites Substances produced by a metabolic process such as the transformation in the body by which energy is made.

Metabolic calcium deposits Calcium formation due to a metabolic process.

Multigym See equipment portfolio.

Muscle identification Self awareness in association with muscle action.

Muscle release The ability to relieve muscles of unwanted tension without conscious thought.

Musculo-skeletal Pertaining to or comprising the skeleton and muscles.

Neuro-muscular co-ordination The control of muscular movement by the brain to perform a given task efficiently.

Negative muscular state A state in which the muscles have the least possible tension yet remain efficient.

Oxygen debt When the demand of the working muscles for oxygen exceeds the supply, thereby incurring a debt.

Oxygen uptake The amount of oxygen that one requires for a given activity taken into the body and utilised for oxidation.

Par Standard according to equality of value.

Palpitation Unduly rapid action of the heart of which the subject is aware.

Peak flow Maximum forced expiratory flow rate as a measure of ventilatory capacity.

Pelvic girdle The pelvis with its attached musculature.

Pelvic floor muscles The deep muscles within the pelvic girdle responsible for the forcing action of the bowel and bladder, etc.

Protocols Designs of measurement used in exercise testing.

Pulse recovery rate The time taken for the post exercise pulse rate to fall to a pre-determined level.

Pressure bandage A series of, usually, three crepe bandages between each of which is a layer of cotton wool. Used to minimise swelling, prevent movement and to relieve pain.

Sacrum The triangular bone at the base of the spine, formed by five fused vertebrae.

Sciatica Inflammation of the sciatic nerve, usually caused by pressure at one or more of its roots in the lower back. This often leads to pain which radiates down the course of the nerve.

Somatotype A system of identifying physique by shape not size.

Static stretch The holding of a position in which a set of muscles are kept under full stretch. Usually for 5 to 10 seconds.

Subscapular Situated below or under the shoulder blade.

Supra-iliac Above or over the crest of the pelvis towards the side.

Supine Lying face upward.

Syndrome A set of symptoms which occur together.

Systolic Pertaining to or produced by the contraction of the heart.

Triceps The muscle that lies at the back of the upper arm, and is responsible in part for extension of the elbow joint.

Tone The normal degree of muscle tension even during periods of muscle stasis.

Volume cylinder This refers to a Peak Flow Meter.

Warm down Used to refer to a period at the end of hard muscular activity, when a few gentle and rhythmical exercises help to restore the normal body chemistry.

Watt A measurement of power. Used in this book it refers to the power and total bodily effort required for a set of load factors.